Prescribed Drugs and tne Alternative Practitioner

DEDICATION

To my wife, Hilary, for her love and support and to all my teachers: may I have the good fortune to recognise them for what they are.

STEPHEN GASCOIGNE
MB., ChB., C.Ac.

Prescribed Drugs
and the
Alternative Practitioner

BATH
ENERGY MEDICINE PRESS

First published in Great Britain by
ENERGY MEDICINE PRESS
An imprint of Ashgrove Press Limited
4 Brassmill Centre, Brassmill Lane
Bath, Avon BA1 3JN

ISBN 1 85398 022 6

First published 1992

Distributors
AcuMedic CENTRE
101-105 CAMDEN HIGH STREET
LONDON NW1 7JN
Tel: 0171-388 5783/6704
Catalogue on Request

Photoset by
Ann Buchan (Typesetters), Middlesex
Printed and bound in Great Britain

CONTENTS

Chapter

	Preface	7
1	Introduction	9
2	Drugs – What they are and how they act	11
3	How to use the book	18
4	Acute disease	32
5	Tricky cases	55
6	Psychoactive drugs	64
7	Cardiovascular system	98
8	Respiratory system	148
9	Gastrointestinal system	180
10	Central nervous system	210
11	Arthritis	242
12	Endocrine	258
13	Dermatology	277
14	Endnotes	293
	Footnotes	294
	Bibliography	295
	Appendix	296
	Sample Letter	297
	General Index	298
	Drug Index	300

ACKNOWLEDGEMENTS

For invaluable help in the process of creation: Hilary Gascoigne, Laurence Gerlis, Hugh McPherson, Arabella Melville and numerous colleges, staff and students of alternative medicine.

PREFACE

I had one main objective when writing this book and this was to provide information about prescribed drugs which practitioners of alternative medicine can use in their practice. This is to enable patients to withdraw conventional medication when appropriate. As patients improve with treatment by alternative medicine then prescribed drugs become unnecessary. I do not intend this, directly at least, for patients and anyone without a professional training should seek to consult a competent practitioner.

The whole area of drug-taking, whether prescribed or 'social', is difficult to come to terms with both individually and as a society. The National Health Service spends over £3 billion per year on drugs and this takes no account of money spent on over-the-counter remedies. Most patients attending for treatment[1] take prescribed drugs and scant attention has been paid to this by practitioners or schools of alternative medicine. There is a hope or wish that the problem will go away, perhaps of its own volition or by someone else taking responsibility.

This is unrealistic. It is time to grasp the nettle and for practitioners to take charge of this aspect of their patient's case. Doctors find it difficult to provide a way since they are primarily the cause of so many drug prescriptions. I know from my own experience that they may have few other skills to help people who are ill and so drugs are their fall-back position. Now this is clearly a difficult area because medical practitioners see themselves very often as being the main providers of health care and the experts in areas such as prescribed drugs. My personal opinion is that patients must be allowed to decide for themselves what is appropriate and what is not. They do this with the help of practitioners – alternative and/or orthodox. Therefore, alternative practitioners must begin to get involved in areas traditionally seen to be the remit of doctors. This means that you have to be well trained in your therapy, responsible in its use and versed in the management of patients taking drugs. There are a few situations where conventional help may be needed but these are uncommon. If patients are to find a way towards health, towards freedom from limitation, towards greater awareness and understanding then this entails movement away from drugs and their consequences.

I do not pretend that it is easy to start thinking of these matters since it can shake the very roots of our belief in Western science, society and medicine. Make no mistake, most of us still hold on emotionally to conventional medicine and conventional systems of thought. Change can be threatening and I know when I teach about drugs there are many reactions to the ideas discussed.

Anger directed at the medical profession, sadness when patient's experiences are retold, guilt at having taken drugs in the past (or having prescribed them!) are just some of the feelings expressed. Although these may be understandable they are not always helpful and merely prevent us getting to grips with the very issues causing them.

We must find our own ways of resolving these difficulties whilst addressing problems of drugs in our patients. I hope this book will help practitioners do this.

I have spent little time arguing the philosophical base of alternative medicine. I have assumed that practitioners are well versed in this and need no discussion here of that nature. I have also assumed that practitioners know of conventional disease labels, their meaning and conventional management and treatment. This is not intended to be a pathology book. That is a major project in its own right.

My personal approach to health and disease is from the direction of Chinese medicine with ideas of suppression, 'cure' and levels of health being those of homoeopathic philosophy.

Have courage in your practice, do not be afraid to ask for help when required but remember that competent, well trained practitioners already have the skills. They may merely lack the knowledge and confidence this book seeks to provide.

1 INTRODUCTION

The use of drugs and chemicals is widespread in our society. There are large sections of the population who rely on such agents to alter their mental, emotional or physical state. Modern medicine is not immune from this and many of us involved in alternative medicine do so as a reaction to this reliance.

Most patients who present for treatment are taking drugs which have been prescribed by a medical practitioner. Many more are taking drugs 'socially'. Cases are therefore complicated as drugs alter symptoms and may lead to further deterioration in health. The regaining of health and the responsibility for one's own condition usually involves the reduction or removal of these chemicals.

It is usually considered that this is the role of the medical profession. I would dispute this. It is the medical profession which is primarily responsible for the drugs taken by patients and for the conventional treatment of disease. Any alternative route will not come from this direction. Just as patients have to take responsibility for their health and their actions, so alternative practitioners have to take responsibility for health matters involving their patients. Prescribed drugs are an important aspect of this.

This book is designed to give information which practitioners can use, with their patients. This can be done alone in many cases, without the need to resort to advice from the orthodox profession. There is no fault with seeking sources of sympathetic information but as many practitioners know orthodox advice may be limiting rather than facilitating.

Drugs do present problems for alternative practitioners and it is an area which has been much neglected in both training and clinical practice. The confusion surrounding the use of drugs and how this affects the practice of medicine can seem almost insurmountable.

Confusion is widespread – patients may not know why they are taking a particular medication or understand its effects and side- effects. Doctors also do not know the full effects of a drug or how it will interact with a patient.

There is simply insufficient information available about the actions of drugs and the effects they have on people or their particular conditions. They are not studied in the same way as homoeopathic remedies, where a substance is given to groups of healthy people and the symptoms experienced are recorded in their entirety – mental, emotional and physical. Drugs are given to people who already have symptoms, for indeterminate periods of time and with no accurate recording of their effects. Clinical trials are performed but no-one is interested in the totality of the symptoms produced by each drug – only in one (usually physical) effect.

In clinical practice patients are prescribed several drugs at the same time. They are not tested in this way, only singly, and although some drug interactions are known I would suggest that many are not.

There is no long term follow-up of patients who take drugs with the specific purpose of checking whether people who take similar drugs for similar diseases develop related conditions later. People are supposed to report adverse reactions to their doctor and these may, or may not, be relayed to the relevant authorities. The Committee for the Safety of Medicines which receives this information only has advisory powers even then.

The result is that no prospective study is carried out and so drug tragedies such as thalidomide, ERALDIN, OPREN continue to occur.

This lack of information and its inevitable confusion pervades the whole area of prescribed drugs and no-one is exempt from its influence. This may help alternative practitioners not to take this personally. The feeling is universal.

2 DRUGS – BACKGROUND

Pharmacology is the study of drugs and for most alternative practitioners it is not necessary to enter into details of their chemical structure and action. Emphasis here will be to relate drugs to case management rather than merely reproduce the conventional information available in orthodox texts.

Pharmacology is a relatively new speciality and only dates from the latter half of the 19th Century. Considering the number of changes which have occurred in drug treatment in that short time it seems surprising that so many people put so much faith in them.

Drugs are defined as, ' . . . any substance which can alter the structure or function of the living organism.'[2]

They are considered to have effects on the underlying physical and chemical processes in the body. There is no thought here, as with orthodox medicine in general, of energetic concepts or mental and emotional spheres of action. The emphasis is on the solid, physical plane.

SUPPRESSION AND SIDE-EFFECTS

Drugs are given according to the principles of Western Medicine and so tend to be suppressive when considered from the energetic viewpoint. That is, they do not 'cure' they merely replace the original condition by another, drug-induced condition which is usually more severe than the original[3]. For detailed information I would refer the reader to *The Science of Homoeopathy* by G. Vithoulkas. The book clearly explains suppression, levels of health and how alternative medicine (in this case homoeopathy) can bring about an improvement.

It is this process which can confuse the alternative practitioner. Instead of seeing the symptoms and condition clearly, there is a picture which may be due only to the drug or (more likely) due to a combination of the drug and the original condition. The study of side-effects can shed some light on what is happening since it may be obvious that many of the patient's symptoms are due to the medication.

The term 'side-effect' can be misleading because it suggests that it is a peripheral action. It is important to understand that all drugs have a particular group of actions specific to that agent. They may express themselves slightly differently in individual cases but these actions cannot be avoided. You cannot separate the constipating action of morphine from its sedating one, you cannot separate the blood pressure lowering effect of betablockers from their effects on circulation producing tiredness and cold extremities. All of these actions are a result of the drug being administered. The fact that one action is the desired effect and another a side-effect is purely an arbitrary decision dependent upon the needs of the moment.

Depending on the study examined, there are 1-40% of patients who experience side-effects when taking drugs. The wide variation in figures reflects the type of data collection used. When it is left to patients to spontaneously report information there are very low levels of reporting. When patients are specifically questioned by trained personnel the numbers rise dramatically. Since the former method is the one routinely used in clinical practice it is clear that a large proportion go unrecorded. Around 8% of all hospital admissions are as a result of side-effects of conventional treatment[4], although some studies suggest higher numbers. The drugs most commonly implicated are antibiotics, aspirin, digoxin, diuretics, heparin, insulin, prednisolone and WARFARIN.

Side-effects are conventionally divided into two types.

Type A reactions are considered to be an increased effect of normal. An example of this would be low blood pressure in someone taking hypotensive drugs. These reactions are 80% of the total and are associated with low mortality although I would estimate that morbidity is high. I would think that most patients who take drugs fall into this category – experiencing side-effects on taking a drug. These may be minor and may diminish with time as the body adjusts itself to the changed situation. Cigarette smoking is a good indication of the initial problems of taking a drug which, with continued use, become less and less until hardly noticed.

Type B reactions are unpredictable. An example of this would be the development of bone marrow disorders with carbimazole. These types of reaction are less common but are associated with higher mortality.

The number of side-effects is dependent on several factors. They are more likely with:

- increasing dose
- multiple drug use
- the very young and elderly
- twice as often in women as men

It is also noted that women are twice as likely as men to die as a result of a drug reaction.

The last two statements may reflect the use of the oral contraceptive pill which is widespread and has powerful effects.

An important consideration here is the route of administration, since certain routes are associated with lower dosages and a lower incidence of side-effects. The routes commonly used in increasing order of severity:

- topical (on the skin, for example)
- inhalation
- enteral: oral/rectal
- injection: intravenous/intramuscular/subcutaneous

In this book I shall mainly be considering the first three routes since injected drugs are rarely seen in outpatient practice.

DEPENDENCE

The term addiction has largely been supplanted by dependence and a distinction is made between physical and psychological forms.

Dependence is the desire to continue taking a drug for its effects. Characteristically, withdrawal symptoms are experienced when the drug is reduced in dose or stopped. 'In physical dependence withdrawal of the drug causes specific symptoms (withdrawal symptoms). . . . Much more common is psychological dependence, in which repeated use of a drug induces a reliance on it for a state of well- being and contentment, but there are no physical withdrawal symptoms if use of the drug is stopped.'[5]

The very fact that drugs have an effect means that they can cause dependence if taken regularly. Stopping them or reducing them may lead to the appearance of symptoms. Energetically this is the release of suppressed symptoms and these have to be dealt with if progress is to continue and further reduction of the drug made possible. The distinction between physical and psychological is not completely realistic since body-mind is a continuum. A combination of manifestations is the usual case.

The appearance of withdrawal symptoms is not inevitable and I have seen people who take very large doses for long periods of time and then stop them with no or little trouble. This is however the exception rather than the rule and the appearance of symptoms with dose reduction is exceedingly common.

PRESCRIBED DRUGS AND THE ALTERNATIVE PRACTITIONER

Here I want to discuss the issues I consider to be of importance when looking at the effects of prescribed drugs.

Drugs will Interfere with the Patient's Condition and hence there may be Confusion in making a Correct Diagnosis. Using an example of migraine, a patient may have headaches on the left side of the head, of a throbbing nature with a hot head and eyes. They occur each time there is an emotional upset and in the week before a period. When drugs are introduced the symptoms change. They may disappear altogether, they may be altered in severity, frequency, time of appearance or nature. This will make the work of the practitioner much more difficult.

It is important to make a diagnosis as the case is seen. The clinical picture will be a combination of the original condition and the drugs. The history of the headaches before they were affected by the drugs may also be relevant.

If the clinical picture has completely altered then the drugs may have to be withdrawn gradually until symptoms reappear, a case taken and a diagnosis made.

Drugs may Interfere with Treatment by Alternative Medicine and so lead to Problems with Treatment and Management. Homoeopaths know that drugs are one of the most powerful causes of antidoting a remedy (that is, reversal of its action or movement towards disease). This at the moment is a particularly Western problem and causes great difficulties. It is a common experience in China and societies where drugs are little used that alternative treatment is very effective.

As Any Drug is Withdrawn then its Effect Becomes Less and Less with Each Reduction in Dosage. Alternative treatment will become more effective and the process become smoother and less complicated. The interference by the drug and the confusion of the clinical picture lessens. This is a helpful situation since movement is continuing towards health.

Since Alternative Treatment Changes the Patient's Condition the Need for the Drugs will Change. As a patient with, for example, hypertension improves and the blood pressure becomes more normal then if the dose of drug is not changed the patient will develop low blood pressure. It is important for any drug to be adjusted in dosage in line with any change in the patient's condition. If this is not done the patient will experience what is essentially an overdose of the prescribed drug.

Any Patient who takes Prescribed Drugs is Implicitly or Explicitly Receiving Treatment from a Conventional Medical Practitioner. When such patients are treated a source of possible conflict has arisen. In an ideal world it would be possible to work with colleagues of every persuasion in helping people regain health and vitality. However, the philosophies of alternative and conventional medicine are contradictory and so there are situations where this is not possible. It is important to avoid the patient becoming a battleground between alternative and conventional medicine. Ultimately the choice of treatment lies with the patient not with the prescriber or indeed with the alternative practitioner.

The very fact that a patient on prescribed drugs is coming for treatment means there is a willingness to change. With explanation of the options available the patient will be in a much better position to decide what they want.

How to deal with the doctor who prescribes the drugs is up to every individual practitioner. I believe that it is courteous to be honest about what is done and, if possible, inform the doctor of what is taking place. This assumes that the patient is in agreement. I always write to GPs at the beginning and end of a course of treatment to outline my approach and the results of treatment. It may be useful for you to do the same, as it seems to be the professional response to treating patients who are also under the care of another practitioner. However, and this is a controversial point, it may not be as simple as this. I know from my own experience and from discussions with other alternative practitioners that doctors can be very hostile to suggestions that patients have alternative treatment, let alone move into areas of drug withdrawal. Doctors tend to react defensively, as they feel threatened by such events. I would encourage you to deal with situations on your own with help from your supervisor or a more experienced practitioner in your own therapy. If this is insufficient to deal with the problem then seek the help of a sympathetic conventionally trained practitioner, ideally one who now practises alternative medicine exclusively but if this is not available then search out GPs who can support you. Do not try to deal with hostile, unsympathetic doctors. Build up a network of people who can help deal with difficult cases in a positive way.

There are no legal restrictions on what an alternative practitioner can do so long as it is within their professional competence and expertise. The only exception to this is that you are not allowed to treat sexually transmitted disease such as gonorrhoea or syphilis (Venereal Diseases Act 1916). You should not do anything you do not feel capable of and should seek advice in those cases. You are not allowed to advertise cures or make outrageous claims but these situations are covered by legislation such as the Trades Descriptions Act.

The responsibility for taking the drug lies with the patient. It should never be or seen to be the case that the patient stops or reduces medication on your instructions. This will open the way for possible legal repercussions. The patient is the person who must decide with the benefit of information and support or help offered by the practitioner. There are clearly restrictions on the actual prescription of drugs but these are of no relevance for alternative practitioners.

ENERGETIC VIEW OF PRESCRIBED DRUGS

There are several consequences, depending on the drug used and the condition of the patient.

Firstly there could be no effect. In this case there is no 'connection' between the drug and the patient's energy. There is no effect on the disease and side-effects do not appear. This situation, although not common, does occur and stopping the drug is easy.

Secondly there may an effect on the patient of various types.

a) The symptoms improve but are replaced by a drug disease and/or by the appearance at some later date of a more serious, deeper disease.

b) The effect may be curative due either to the 'placebo' effect or because the drug given is actually the appropriate remedy in terms of energetic medicine.

This latter case is unusual and one example would be the very high success rate seen with the use of platinum for testicular and ovarian tumours. It has been known for many years that the homoeopathic remedy PLATINA (platinum) is indicated in some cases of such tumours. This is an example of conventional medicine stumbling across the appropriate energetic remedy by chance.

The 'placebo' effect is the other way in which symptoms may improve in a curative way, due to the healing power of the doctor. Do not underestimate this ability. Doctors have a high status in our society, particularly surgeons, and the associated power may have a healing effect.

c) The last situation is when the patient's energy is over-whelmed by the drug. Severe disease or death is the result.

There are no other possibilities.

These conclusions can be drawn according to the principles of energetic medicine and the laws of healing. It is beyond the scope of this book to outline these in detail but I would refer the interested reader to textbooks of homoeopathic philosophy as well as texts of Chinese Medicine.

Chinese medicine itself provides a model of subtle energetic anatomy and physiology which may give insights into the actions of drugs. One of the difficulties here is to predict what may happen when patients take drugs – will they affect blood, lung, kidney and so on?

Chinese medicine outlines the energetic qualities of herbs, their energetic functions and the organs affected. With a deep understanding of the principles of Chinese medicine it may be possible to extend this to an energetic account of drugs' actions. This will be of immense benefit to practitioners in uderstanding the effect of drugs on patients and how best to mitigate the worst of their harmful actions.

It is beyond the scope of this book to do this. It is my hope that some time in the future such information can be provided.

3 HOW TO USE THE BOOK

Many practitioners ask how to know the result of drug withdrawal. There is a great fear, amongst practitioners and patients, of dire consequences. This is not the case in the vast majority of situations.

I have developed a way of classifying drugs which accords with priniciples of alternative healing and the direction of 'cure'. The alternative view of a human being, considering the perspective of energy ('qi' in Chinese Medicine, 'vital force' in homoeopathy and so on) is that there are interconnected levels. There is a natural hierarchy of levels and organs within those levels so that it is possible in any particular case to decide on the depth of disease.

Therefore, there are considered to be mental, emotional and physical levels, with the physical being the outermost. 'Cure' is the movement of pathology out of the body from mental to physical. Disease is the movement of pathology into the body from the physical. It is clear to anyone who studies medicine and sees patients that alternative medicine tends to lead to 'cure' and orthodox medicine tends to lead to disease.

So when you deal with a patient who takes prescribed drugs it is important to take these levels into account. In this way it is possible to determine the effects of treatment – 'curative' or suppressive – and to decide upon which drugs it is safest to deal with and in which order, if it is a case of multiple prescription.

The following classification has been developed which can be applied to help decide on the approach to take.

Drug Category

CATEGORY I
Drugs taken on an Occasional Basis for the Relief of Symptoms

This is the simplest situation involving drugs. Here are the minor analgesics of aspirin and paracetamol, antacids and any drug which is taken on a symptomatic basis. These cause the practitioner very few problems. Clearly as the symptoms improve there is no further need to take the medication.

I would include antibiotics here because they are usually

used for minor, self-limiting illness and energetically their effect is one of symptomatic relief rather than 'cure'.

CATEGORY II
Drugs which pose No or Little Threat to Life if Discontinued

I would not, naturally, consider this an advisable thing to do in most cases but I use it as an indication of the strength of the drugs categorised here.

Here can be considered most cases of tranquilliser prescription, anti-inflammatory agents, asthma drugs, treatments for migraine, skin conditions and so on. These cases form the bulk of the work of an alternative medicine outpatient practice.

The drug can be withdrawn or stopped with relative ease if the underlying condition is treated at the same time. According to ideas of levels as discussed above, the drugs used to treat emotional disorders would be dealt with before those used to treat physical disorders.

CATEGORY III
Drugs which cannot be stopped suddenly when used Long Term

Here are drugs such as cortisone, antiepileptic drugs and hypotensive agents such as betablockers and clonidine. Sudden cessation may cause death or severe illness.

The approach to each of these is covered in detail in the relevant sections. With care, in selected cases, they may be withdrawn as improvement in the patient's condition begins to occur.

In terms of levels this category applies to drugs which are used for severe physical disease.

CATEGORY IV
Drugs with Powerful Effects Particularly in the Mental and Emotional Spheres

The drugs I am thinking of here are the major psychoactive agents such as LARGACTIL, SERENACE, MELLERIL, DRO-LEPTAN, antipsychotic drugs in general and lithium compounds. Here we have moved into the mental level of the person and so the effect of these drugs is extremely profound.

These are given for conditions such as schizophrenia, psychoses, delusional states, manic depression and major psychological illnesses. They are characterised by lack of insight and bizarre behaviour. The drugs suppress these serious emotional and mental symptoms.

If such patients are treated or the dosage reduced there may be a return of these symptoms. Unless there are adequate facilities and support a situation may arise which is unmanageable. In the context of an out-patient practice such treatment is inappropriate.

Typically symptoms reappear with full force some 4 to 6 weeks after medication has been stopped. The fact that lack of insight is a major feature means that the patient is no longer in control. In-patient care may be necessary and unless this is available I would urge therapists to consider very carefully before even starting such treatment.

Since alternative medicine in the West is still in a relatively weak position the consequences of such action, unless it is well considered and in the right situation, could be disastrous for ourselves as well as the patient.

CATEGORY V
Drugs which are Essential to keep the Patient Alive

This is actually a small proportion of the total. They are cardiac agents used in particular arrhythmias and replacement of hormones in endocrine deficiency such as hypothyroidism, diabetes mellitus, diabetes insipidus and insufficiency of the adrenal cortex.

If these substances are stopped then the patient will die. The length of time before this occurs is dependent upon the actual condition.

The patient can still be treated whilst these drugs are taken but the dosage must be maintained unless there are specific reasons for change based on monitoring or investigations. Monitoring is very important here and has to be done in conjunction with a doctor.

These categories are not rigid and it may be that a drug may appear in another group because of its dosage, length of treatment or the individual patient. For example, if laxatives are taken regularly every day they would be in category II. In some cases of tranquilliser prescription and asthma drugs the effects are more severe and they would then be more appropriate in category III. However, use this as a general guide.

DRUG INFORMATION

I have listed in the reference sections every drug I consider to be in common usage in outpatient clinical practice. These are the drugs most practitioners will encounter in everyday work. I have omitted more unusual medications.

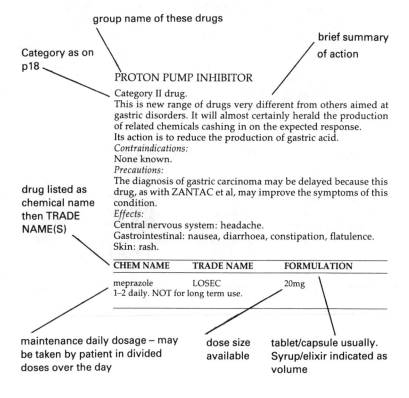

group name of these drugs

brief summary of action

Category as on p18

PROTON PUMP INHIBITOR
Category II drug.
This is new range of drugs very different from others aimed at gastric disorders. It will almost certainly herald the production of related chemicals cashing in on the expected response.
Its action is to reduce the production of gastric acid.
Contraindications:
None known.
Precautions:
The diagnosis of gastric carcinoma may be delayed because this drug, as with ZANTAC et al, may improve the symptoms of this condition.
Effects:
Central nervous system: headache.
Gastrointestinal: nausea, diarrhoea, constipation, flatulence.
Skin: rash.

drug listed as chemical name then TRADE NAME(S)

CHEM NAME	TRADE NAME	FORMULATION
meprazole	LOSEC	20mg
1–2 daily. NOT for long term use.		

maintenance daily dosage – may be taken by patient in divided doses over the day

dose size available

tablet/capsule usually. Syrup/elixir indicated as volume

There are many instances where patients would probably not actually take drugs if they knew of their effects. Consent to treatment can only be considered valid if this is informed consent. I would hope that patients can increase their knowledge of drugs so that they make a genuinely informed decision as to whether they want to take them or not. Decisions of such importance must never be left solely to the practitioner.

General Instructions Applicable to All Drugs

No drug should be given to a person who is sensitive to that or a related substance.

Close monitoring of patients under *Special Precautions* means that patients should have regular contact with their GP or prescribing doctor. This does not mean that patients should be given repeat prescriptions and told to make an appointment in 12 months time. It is certainly true to say that many patients take drugs which are prescribed routinely, even over long periods of time, with little in the way of regular checks as to safety, effectiveness, hazards or even continuing need. There are many drugs which the manufacturers indicate require certain monitoring to be done in cases of chronic use but in clinical practice this infrequently occurs. Drugs such as diuretics, anticonvulsants, hormone replacement therapy at the menopause, lithium compounds are just a few which immediately spring to mind.

Many drugs are hazardous when used in pregnancy or lactation. Assume that all may be harmful unless proved otherwise. It is not good practice to take drugs at such times.

Any drug which causes drowsiness, sedation, tiredness, dizziness and so on may affect driving and the operation of machinery. Patients should be specifically told of this. Alcohol and other sedative drugs aggravate these effects.

Side-effects are generally taken from conventional texts with some additions or comments of my own. I would not assume that these are complete. If a patient takes a drug and develops a certain symptom or group of symptoms then it may well be that the drug is responsible. If the symptom disappears when the drug is stopped this would seem to be confirmation. So do not view lists here as the final word.

Throughout the book I have listed these as 'Effects' rather than 'Side-effects' since they are an integral part of the action of a drug. It is impossible to separate these. To arbitrarily call one the main action and the others 'side-effects' seems to add to the confusion and is in any case misleading.

I have not specifically mentioned interactions for several reasons. Although there are some specific ones which do exist my feeling is that they are commoner than is generally realised. It is not good practice even in conventional circles to give more drugs than is absolutely necessary to minimise the risks of interactions. I tend to look at drugs in terms of their effects and if the patient is taking two drugs which have similar effects then assume that the danger to that patient is increased. This may or may not be seen as an 'interaction'.

I have described case histories at intervals as a way of giving a practical picture of the approach it is possible to take.

Note

Finally, I do not intend any of this to be used by people who are not professionally trained in a form of alternative medicine. I would urge anyone without that training to consult a professional rather than 'go it alone'. Even with training there may be circumstances where liason and supervision are necessary either from a doctor or another practitioner. I would hope that practitioners know their own limitations and seek help where they are confronted by cases outside their experience. It is professionally and legally indefensible to attempt to treat such conditions.

I have indicated in the Preface my views on this. I would encourage you to take personal responsibility for such matters as they affect your patients because it may well be that no-one else is or is able to do so. Seek conventional help if you must but there may be other sources of support not so restrictive or potentially hostile.

FACTORS IN DRUG REDUCTION

How to deal specifically with drugs taken by the patient? There are certain guidelines which can be applied to each case to help with this process and to minimise the adverse effects.

Any Alteration in Dosage may Result in Exacerbation of Symptoms The drug is used to 'control' symptoms. These must be dealt with and as drugs are withdrawn may have to be considered as part of the total picture to be treated. Reduction in dosage must be slow since a flare-up which is unmanageable should be avoided if possible.

Reduce the Dose when the Patient's Condition Starts to

Improve In this way the confidence of the patient is gained, the correct diagnosis and treatment are confirmed and the release of suppressed symptoms will not overwhelm the patient.

I never treat a patient at the first visit and reduce the drugs at the same time. This is to prevent a confusing situation where I am unsure if symptoms which then appear are due to my treatment or to the drug withdrawal. I treat several times, depending upon the case and the drug involved, before moving onto drug withdrawal. In this way different factors are separated and can be clearly addressed one at a time.

Diagnosis is Vital Although it is interesting and even helpful to study drugs, this is the main consideration. A thorough knowledge of the practitioner's therapy is paramount. By diagnosis I mean selection of the appropriate remedy by a homoeopath, pattern of disharmony by a practitioner of Chinese medicine, and so on.

The hope for the patient is through the therapy you practise. It is no good pushing the patient into reducing drugs unless they have begun to improve. They will only improve through the therapy you practise and the help you can offer. Have faith in your therapy, since increasing competence in this will necessarily lead you to deal with more complicated cases effectively. You will find that effective treatment by alternative medicine merely makes the need for the prescription of drugs unnecessary.

Ask about the Original Condition for which the Patient Received the Drugs This may give an indication of the severity of the condition at that time. Some patients do not know why they are taking a drug – they were not told, they have forgotten or they were given several drugs together for different conditions.

Some drugs are prescribed inappropriately by a medical practitioner and this is always something which should be borne in mind. Do not assume that conventional diagnoses and treatment are always correct or if the diagnosis is correct that the treatment is rational. An alarming number of conventional medical diagnoses are in fact mistaken.

For example, if a patient was originally given a major tranquilliser such as LARGACTIL for a delusional state it would be a very different situation than if it were given for mild anxiety.

Severity of the Drugs See classification on page 18. In general the stronger the drug the more severe the patient's condition.

Duration of the Treatment Clearly 6 weeks is much less of a problem than 16 years. I have known patients who have taken very powerful drugs for a long time and then stopped them with no or little problems but I think this is the exception rather than the rule. The longer the patient has taken a prescribed drug then the more likely there is to be dependence (this actually occurs after one or two months of continual use in most cases) and the more likely there are to be problems when the drug is reduced.

Dose of the Drug In the details of each drug the dosages prescribed in each situation are listed. Compare this with the dosage the patient is taking. Is this low, medium or high? A low dosage is clearly easier to deal with than a high dosage. However bear in mind that there is individual variation and some patients have severe problems reducing some drugs which are taken in very low dosage. If in doubt merely reduce very slowly and monitor carefully.

Other Drugs Used It is much easier to deal with one drug than with several. There are interactions between them, each has different effects and it can be more difficult to thread a way out of them.

With Multiple Prescriptions Reduce the most Powerful Drug First It is important not to be left with a situation where the less powerful drugs have been stopped and there is the large hurdle of dealing with a very powerful agent alone.

The less powerful drugs can be used as support whilst it is reduced and the patient's health will recover quicker once that is dealt with. This is in line with homoeopathic philosophy – Hering's Law of Cure. It is important to remove first the drugs which affect deeper levels the most and so go through from Category V to I in the classification above. The only proviso is that drugs which are used for life threatening disorders such as insulin in diabetes mellitus may, in some cases, have to be left alone and so milder drugs would then be reduceed.

This may be the opposite approach to that of many conventional doctors who are involved with drug withdrawal. However from experience it is the most fruitful.

Which is the most powerful drug? Usually the one with the most severe effects. Check these in the reference sections and I have indicated which category they fit into (I, II, III, IV or V).

Usually more powerful drugs are added in sequence by conventional doctors, so drugs can be dealt with in the reverse order to that in which they were given. This is by no means invariable but can be a useful guide.

Assess the Strength of the Patient's Energy If this is weak then the condition is more serious, the effects of withdrawal will be more pronounced and the process needs to be much slower. You may need to treat the patient for many months before their condition improves to the point where drug withdrawal is possible.

Underlying Disease – Serious or not Serious? In life-threatening disease or those conditions with the potential to become so the therapist should obviously tread much more warily. The support and help of others may be needed. In terms of the classification above. Drugs in Category V are usually those used for life threatening disease.

Support for the Patient The original situation required the use of drugs to suppress symptoms. Is this now the time for these to be released and transformed? This is particularly true in the case of psychological disorders. If there is little support at home then the release of suppressed emotional and mental symptoms may not be manageable.

It may be that other help may be required for the patient, such as counselling, psychotherapy, massage, healing and so on. Certainly the more serious the case the more likely it is that a multiple approach will be helpful. In such cases ensure that one person has overall responsibility for the management since patients can become lost in the midst of several practitioners.

Practitioner's Practice Patients who reduce their drugs, depending on the individual case and the drug involved, often need a lot of support. The practitioner may only visit a town once a week or fortnight and not be available for advice or support. The patient may feel very isolated during what can be a very difficult time.

Support for the Therapist It is not sufficient to talk about support for the patient without considering the other side of the equation. It is important that each therapist works out their own system of self-help, professional support and advice. I would consider as a minimum regular supervision sessions, adequate rest and relaxation as well as frequent peer group meetings for mutual support. Treatment for the practitioner may also be required.

I know from personal experience that treating patients uses a lot of energy and personal resources. It is essential that you monitor your own performance and health and take measures to minimise problems.

GENERAL RULES FOR DRUG REDUCTION

Reduce the drug slowly after initial improvement has been obtained. This is mandatory for corticosteroids, betablockers and clonidine – Category III – but is in fact advisable in the vast majority of cases. In essence the approach is to replace the drug by your treatment. Therefore, you must wait until the patient's condition has begun to improve. Otherwise removal of the drugs will lead to a flare-up of the unresolved problem.

The actual reduction can be done by taking the drug less often, splitting the dose or asking the doctor to prescribe a smaller dose. By checking the details of each drug it may be that a smaller dose is available either by the same or another manufacturer. Most tablets will split. In the case of capsules it is possible to separate the two halves, divide the powder or granules and replace in the capsule. It is not wise for people to just take the powder, because of the taste.

The way a drug is reduced in dosage also depends on how often it is taken each day. With once daily dosage this is simple.

What to do when drugs are taken twice, three or even four times each day? Try to keep a smooth dosage over the day so if the drugs are taken morning and evening reduce each one in turn rather than stopping one and then moving on to the other.

In the case of drugs taken three or four times each day, after gradual reductions of each dosage I usually stop the middle-of-the-day ones first. In this way the evening and morning dosages, which are taken after a long interval, are left until last.

I would emphasise that flexibility is required here and changes may be made depending upon the situation, the patient, the drug and the condition.

It is generally possible to reduce more quickly if the condition is mild, the dose is low and the duration of treatment short.

Worked Examples of Multiple Prescription

1. Patient with asthma:

   INTAL INHALER two doses four times daily.

prednisolone 5mg daily.
VENTOLIN INHALER two doses four times daily.
BECOTIDE INHALER two doses three times daily.

This is a common situation seen in asthmatic patients. A combination of inhalers and tablets. There is an oral corticosteroid (prednisolone) and inhaled bronchodilator (VENTOLIN), corticosteroid (BECOTIDE) and mast cell stabiliser (INTAL).

The most powerful ones here will be the corticosteroids with the oral having more effects than the inhaled form. Of the other two, although INTAL is not listed as producing many side-effects it will mask the true picture. It prevents the development of the symptoms. In actual fact many patients say that INTAL has no or very little effect. If this is the case then it can be stopped first – sudden withdrawal has no problems.

If a large allergic component is suspected then it must be withdrawn gradually after the corticosteroids have been removed. The bronchodilator can be reduced at a rate to suit the patient. It can be taken when required rather than all the time no matter the situation.

Order of withdrawal:

- INTAL?
- prednisolone
- BECOTIDE
- INTAL?
- VENTOLIN

2. Patient with pains in the chest following a heart attack 2 years ago.

The amitryptiline and VALIUM were added in the last year because of difficulties with a close relationship.

FRUSENE 1 daily.
amitryptiline 25mg at night.
VALIUM 5mg twice daily.
isosorbide mononitrate 10mg three times daily.

Here there is a mixture of medication for a physical problem and emotional state. In general it is better to clear up the deeper levels first and so deal with the tranquilliser (VALIUM) and antidepressant (amitryptiline). Of the two, antidepressants are very powerful and have many more severe effects than minor tranquillisers.

In the case of the diuretic (FRUSENE) and nitrate (isosorbide mononitrate) it is better gradually to change the nitrate over to symptomatic use, i.e. only take when necessary. Then reduce the diuretic slowly before the nitrate is finally stopped. There may be the appearance of oedema or fluid retention when this done. This is on the physical level – discharge of 'fluid' on the emotional level may occur in the form of emotional upset, weeping and so on.

Order of withdrawal:

- change isosorbide dinitrate to symptomatic use, i.e. Category I
- amitryptiline
- VALIUM
- FRUSENE
- isosorbide dinitrate

3. Patient of 83 years with hypertension, BP 150/75. Has felt tired, poor memory, lack of concentration since put on tablets for dizziness 6 months ago. She has had treatment for her blood pressure for several years.

She has taken paracetamol since an operation for hiatus hernia left her with a painful scar some 20 or so years ago.

TENORMIN LS 50mg three daily.
bendrofluazide 5mg daily.
paracetamol 500mg two four times daily.
STEMETIL 5mg three times daily.

This is a common situation particularly in the elderly: multiple prescriptions with the addition of extra drugs as other symptoms appear. It is not uncommon to see elderly patients on 4,5, 6 or even more different drugs.

The first comment to make is that the blood pressure is LOW given her age and the dose of TENORMIN (betablocker) is more than the recommended amount.

A medium potency diuretic (bendrofluazide) adds to the hypotensive effect of the betablocker. Paracetamol is an analgesic although the length of time this patient has taken it is considerable.

STEMETIL is a phenothiazine tranquilliser (related to LARGACTIL and other antipsychotic agents) and is used for psychoses or, as here, for dizziness.

The dizziness was almost certainly due to the low blood pressure brought on by the overdosing of the hypotensive agents. So stop the STEMETIL first. After a short period of irritability she was much more alert.

Reduce the TENORMIN LS to twice daily. This led to a small increase in blood pressure which was OK for her age.

The drugs to deal with later if it is possible to stop the TENORMIN LS are bendrofluazide and then the paracetamol
Order of withdrawal:

- STEMETIL
- TENORMIN LS
- bendrofluazide
- paracetamol

In this situation it was only possible to reduce the TENORMIN LS to 50mg daily. The blood pressure stabilised at 170/95, she felt well, was alert and could manage her daily life again.

In many elderly people it may not be possible to stop drugs completely, particularly if they have come to alternative medicine late and drug treatment has been long-term. Other factors such as diet, exercise and relaxation may also not be as amenable to change as in younger age groups.

4. Patient of 70 years with a diagnosis of Parkinson's disease. Her medication was:

selegiline 5mg twice daily
SINEMET 110 4 daily
orphenadrine 50mg twice daily
PROTHIADEN 75mg at night

Here there is a situation of an antidepressant prescribed with 3 types of anti-Parkinsonian drugs. If you check the details of PROTHIADEN you will see that it is a tricyclic antidepressant. This should never be prescribed with mono-amine oxidase inhibitors because of the risk of adverse reactions such as hypertension. However selegiline is such a drug.

Also the side-effects of PROTHIADEN are very heating (constipation, insomnia, anxiety, dry mouth, rapid heart rate) as are the side-effects of orphenadrine. Therefore we have a case here where there are 3 drugs reacting with each other. The patient's main symptoms were those of dry mouth, shaking inside, anxiety, tremor!

PROTHIADEN is the dangerous one in this situation and must be stopped as soon as possible, certainly within one week. Patients can die if they take a tricyclic antidepressant and a mono-amine oxidase inhibitor together.

Of the others SINEMET is the most powerful acting drug with the remaining two being of little distinction.

So the order of withdrawal is:

- PROTHIADEN
- SINEMET
- orphenadrine or selegiline

LIASON WITH DOCTORS

There are many situations where this is not necessary, given that the expertise and knowledge of the practitioner is satisfactory. I would consider help from a conventionally trained practitioner essential for the following conditions:

- drugs which are essential for life e.g. insulin, cardiac drugs for arrhythmias, replacement with thyroid hormone, vasopressin, corticosteroids in cases of insufficiency of the adrenal cortex (Addison's disease) – Category V
- life-threatening conditions – Category V
- conditions requiring in-patient therapy.
- conditions with legal restrictions on treatment (sexually transmitted diseases).

I have included in the Appendix some examples of how to phrase letters to other practitioners, be these orthodox or alternative. It is never good practice to pass messages via patients. Contact the other professional directly; a letter is the professional way to do this. It is fine to ring up other practitioners but I would be careful of doing this to an orthodox practitioner unless you are sure of your position and envisage a sympathetic response.

4   ACUTE DISEASE

Acute illnesses are commonly the infectious diseases of ortho-dox medicine. They are often treated with antibiotics, although conventionally only bacterial illnesses should be prescribed these drugs. Antibiotics in reality are commonly used for mild disease and inappropriately in the case of viral disease.

How to manage this situation?

If a patient comes for treatment with an acute febrile illness and is taking an antibiotic then alternative treatment can be instituted as usual.

Make an assessment as to the vitality of the patient and the severity of the condition.

If the patient is usually quite well and has a relatively mild condition the antibiotic can be stopped immediately and the patient treated as if the case were uncomplicated. There will be few problems of suppression to deal with and the patient can be seen every other day or whenever necessary.

There is the question here of development of resistance to the antibiotic. This is the rationale behind telling patients to complete the whole course of treatment.

There have been marked changes in recent years of the recommended length of time that antibiotics should be taken. This is especially obvious with urinary tract infections. When I qualified in the mid-70s, seven or even ten days of treatment was the rule. Now you see prescriptions of three single doses.

However the main problem is with the patient NOT the bacteria. Further harm to the immune system is prevented by removing the antibiotics and alternative treatment will strengthen people so that the underlying imbalance is rectified.

If the patient has had courses of antibiotics previously for a similar or related condition then it can be assumed the problem is more long-standing.

In the case of a patient with strong energy then assess the situation after treatment. If the patient is beginning to recover by the second visit the antibiotics can be stopped with safety. Treatment can be continued and the patient will need to have regular sessions after the acute episode in view of the history of recurrent illnesses.

In the case of a patient with weak energy then it may well be that removal of the antibiotic will cause a flare-up which cannot be dealt with adequately. Try to alleviate the acute symptoms as far as possible, avoid interfering with the antibiotics and when the acute illness is over treat the underlying condition. In this way the acute manifestations are not exacerbated by the release of suppressions when drugs are withdrawn.

It is helpful to make it clear to patients that acute illnesses can and are treated by alternative medicine, that acute illnesses occurring in patients having regular treatment are often related to the chronic condition and that antibiotics may deplete the patient's energy causing problems to be dealt with at a later date.

The final situation which may be seen with regard to antibiotics is when they are prescribed on a regular basis for conditions such as acne, urinary tract infections and respiratory conditions. Here they can be dealt with as for any drug which is taken continually. Obviously, you should bear in mind the original condition and consider the need for regular monitoring of the infective state.

SUMMARY

Category I — most cases of antibiotic prescription
Category II — those cases such as acne, chronic urinary tract infection where antibiotics are given long term
Category V — life threatening disease such as meningitis or AIDS

Antibacterials

PENICILLIN

This is a very commonly used antibiotic. It may produce allergic reactions (at least in 1% of patients) including anaphylaxis and death.
Effects:
Central nervous system: dizziness.
Gastrointestinal: nausea, vomiting, indigestion, diarrhoea, black hairy tongue, hepatitis.
Colitis may occur so diarrhoea must be viewed with suspicion.
Urogenital: nephritis.
Blood: neutropenia, agranulocytosis, pancytopenia, thrombocytopenia.
Allergic: urticaria, sore throat, fever, chills, oedema, joint pains, bruising or bleeding, anaphylaxis.

CHEM NAME	TRADE NAME	FORMULATION
amoxycillin	ALMODAN	250mg, 500mg, 125mg/5ml, 250mg/5ml
	AMORAM	250mg, 500mg, 125mg/5ml, 250mg/5ml
	AMOXIL	250mg, 500mg, 125mg/5ml, 250mg/5ml 125mg/1.25ml (children)
	GALENAMOX	250mg, 500mg, 125 and 250mg/5ml

250-500mg three times daily.
Children: half adult dose.
Used as higher dosages (750mg twice daily) for severe or recurrent otitis media.

	AMOXIL 3G SACHET	3G

For severe respiratory infection, acute urinary tract infection. 3G twice daily. 2 doses only in some cases of urinary tract infection.

	AMOXIL 750mg SACHET SF	750mg

Used in otitis media.
Under 3 years of age not recommended, 3-10 years 750mg twice daily for 2 days.

	AUGMENTIN	250mg with 125mg clavulanic acid

1-2 three times daily for up to 14 days.

	AUGMENTIN JUNIOR	125mg with 62mg clavulanic acid/5ml

Children: 6-12 years 5ml three times daily for up to 14 days.

	AUGMENTIN PAED.	125mg with 31mg clavulanic acid/5ml

Children: under 3 months not recommended, 3-9 months 2.5ml half-strength, 9 months- 2years 5ml half-strength, 2-6 years 5ml. All three times daily for up to 14 days.
Clavulanic acid is a betalactamase inhibitor. Betalactamase is produced by some bacteria which are therefore penicillin resistant. Clavulanic acid seems to increase the gastrointestinal effects of amoxycillin.

ampicillin	AMFIPEN	250mg, 500mg, 125mg/5ml, 250mg/5ml
	PENBRITIN	250mg, 500mg, 125mg/5ml, 125mg/1.25ml (children)
	PENBRITIN FORTE	250mg/5ml

| | VIDOPEN | 250mg, 500mg, 125mg and 250mg/5ml |

250-1G four times daily.
Children: half adult dose.

| | MAGNAPEN | 250mg with 250mg flucloxacillin |
| | | 125mg with 125mg flucloxacillin/5ml |

1 capsule or 10ml four times daily.
Children: under 2 years quarter adult dose, under 10 years 5ml four times daily.
With the addition of a penicillinase resistant antibiotic.
Ampicillin must never be used in cases of glandular fever because of the high incidence of rashes associated with its use in this condition.

bacampicillin   AMBAXIN   400mg
1-2 two or three times daily.
Children: under 5 years not recommended, over 5 years half tablet three times daily.

benzathine   PENIDURAL   222mg/5ml
penicillin
10ml three to four times daily.
Children: half adult dose.

                   PENIDURAL   115mg/ml
                   ORAL DROPS
Children up to 5 years: 1-2 droppersful three to four times daily.

carfecillin   UTICILLIN   500mg
1-2 three times daily.
Children: Not under 2 years, 2-10 years 30-60mg/Kg daily.
Usually used for urinary tract infections.

ciclacillin   CALTHOR   250mg, 500mg
1-2G daily.
Children: under 2 months not recommended, over 2 months 50-100mg/Kg daily.

cloxacillin   ORBENIN   250mg, 500mg, 125mg/5ml
500mg four times daily.
Children: under 2 years one quarter adult dose, over 2 years half adult dose.

flucloxacillin   FLOXAPEN   250mg, 500mg, 125mg/5ml
                   FLOXAPEN FORTE   250mg/5ml
                   LADROPEN   250mg, 500mg
                   STAFOXIL   250mg, 500mg
                   STAPHLIPEN   250mg, 500mg
250mg four times daily.
Children: under 2 years quarter adult dose; 2-10 years half adult dose.

penicillin V   APSIN V.K.   250mg, 125mg/5ml,

	250mg/5ml
DISTAQUAINE V-K	250mg, 125mg/5ml, 250mg/5ml
STABILLIN V-K	250mg, 62.5mg, 125mg/5ml, 250mg/5ml
V-CIL-K	250mg, 125mg/5ml, 250mg/5ml

125-250mg four to six times daily.
Children: under 1 year 62.5mg, 1-5 years 125mg, over 5 years 125-250mg. All four times daily.

phenethicillin	BROXIL	250mg, 125mg/5ml

250mg four times daily.
Children: under 2 years quarter adult dose, over 2 years half adult dose.

pivampicillin	PONDOCILLIN	500mg, 175mg/5ml, 175mg sachets

1 tablet or 15ml or 3 sachets twice daily.
Children: under 1 year 40-60mg/Kg daily, 1-5 years 10-15ml or 2-3 sachets daily, 6-10 years 15-20ml or 3-4 sachets daily.

	MIRAXID	125mg with 100mg pivmecillinam
	MIRAXID PAED. SUSP.	62.5mg with 46.2mg pivmecillinam (sachets)

2-4 tablets twice daily.
Children: under 6 years 1-2 sachets twice daily, 6-10 years 1 tablet or 2-3 sachets twice daily, over 10 years same as adult.

	MIRAXID 450	250mg with 200mg pivmecillinam
	PONDOCILLIN PLUS	250mg with 200mg pivmecillinam

1-2 twice daily.
Children: under 10 not recommended, over ten 1 twice daily.

pivmecillinam	SELEXID	200mg, 100mg (sachets)

2 tablets or 4 sachets three times daily for recurrent bacteria in the urine.
Other infections 1.2-2.4G daily for 14 days.
Children: under 40Kg 20-40mg/Kg daily for urinary tract infection and 30-60mg/Kg for others. Over 40Kg as adult.

talampicillin	TALPEN	250mg, 125mg/5ml

250mg three times daily.
Children: under 2 years 3-7 mg/Kg, over 2 years 125mg. Both three times daily.

CEPHALOSPORIN

Another commonly used antibiotic group. There is often cross sensitivity between these and the penicillins.
Effects:
General: drowsiness.
Central nervous system: headache, dizziness, increased muscle tone.
Psychological: hyperactivity, anxiety, insomnia, confusion.
Gastrointestinal: stomatitis, diarrhoea, nausea, vomiting, indigestion, abdominal cramps, irritation of mouth or tongue, jaundice, colitis, abnormal liver function tests, hepatitis.
Urogenital: nephritis, changes in renal function, haematuria, vaginitis.
Allergic: urticaria, fever, sore throat, itching, joint pains, anaphylaxis.
Blood disorders: agranulocytosis, leucopenia, eosinophilia, thrombocytopenia.

CHEM NAME	TRADE NAME	FORMULATION
cefaclor	DISTACLOR	250mg, 125mg/5ml, 250mg/5ml

250mg three time daily. Maximum 4G daily.
Children: under 1 year quarter adult dose, 1-5 years half adult dose, over 5 years same as adult.

cefadroxil	BAXAN	500mg, 125mg/5ml, 250mg/5ml, 500mg/5ml

500mg-1G twice daily.
Children: under 1 year 25mg/Kg daily, 1-6 years 250mg twice daily, over 6 years 500mg twice daily.

cefuroxime	ZINNAT	125mg, 250mg

250mg twice daily. Severe infections 500mg twice daily.
Children: under 5 years not recommended, over 5 years 125mg twice daily. 250mg twice daily in otitis media.

cephalexin	CEPOREX	250mg, 500mg, 1G, 125mg/5ml, 250mg/5ml 500mg/5ml, 125mg/1.25ml(children)
	KEFLEX	250mg, 500mg, 125mg/5ml, 250mg/5ml

1-2G daily.
Children: under 3 months 62.5mg-125mg twice daily, 4 months to 2 years 250-500mg daily, 3-6 years 500mg-1G daily, 6-12 years 1-2G daily.
This may cause a reversible toxic psychosis.

cephradine   VELOSEF   250mg, 500mg, 250mg/5ml
1-2G daily, maximum 4G daily.
Children: 25-50mg/Kg daily. For otitis media 75-100mg/Kg daily.
Maximum 4G daily.

NITROFURAN

This is a small group usually used for urinary tract infections.
They may be given long-term (over many years) for some cases
of resistant infection.
Contraindications:
Marked renal impairment.
Precautions:
Lung reactions can occur and these may be fatal. The drug must
be stopped immediately if any respiratory symptoms occur.
This is particularly relevant in the case of long-term therapy.
Monitoring of liver function should be undertaken regularly
with long-term use since jaundice and hepatitis can occur. Liver
dysfunction may be lifethreatening and deaths have occurred.
Peripheral neuropathy as evidenced by parasthesiae can occur
and may be life-threatening. The development of such a symptom requires immediate withdrawal of the drug. The risk of
such a complication is increased by the presence of underlying
disease such as anaemia, diabetes mellitus, renal impairment
and vitamin B deficiency.
Effects:
General: drowsiness.
Central nervous system: peripheral neuropathy (may be severe
and irreversible), vertigo, dizziness, headache.
Respiratory: acute reactions include fever, chills, cough, chest
pain, dyspnoea. Chronic reactions include malaise, dyspnoea,
cough.
Gastrointestinal: nausea, anorexia, vomiting, abdominal pain,
diarrhoea, jaundice, hepatitis, pancreatitis.
Urogenital: infection of the urinary tract by resistant organisms
may occur. These are often more dangerous than the original
organism in terms of the possibility of damage. Brown discolouration of urine.
Skin: rashes, itching, alopecia.
Blood disorders: agranulocytosis, leucopenia, granulocytopenia, haemolytic anaemia, thrombocytopenia, megaloblastic
anaemia, aplastic anaemia.

CHEM NAME	TRADE NAME	FORMULATION
nitrofurantoin	FURADANTIN	50mg, 100mg, 25mg/5ml
	MACRODANTIN	50mg, 100mg

50-100mg four times daily. Long term usage 50-100mg daily.
Children: under 1 month not recommended, 1 month-2 years 12.5mg,
2½-6 years 25mg, 6-11 years 50mg, 11-14 years 50-100mg. All four times
daily. For long-term usage quarter to half of above doses once daily.

TETRACYCLINE

This group is commonly used for minor infections of the upper
respiratory and urinary tracts. It is used for acne where it is
given in smaller doses over a period of several months.
Contraindications:
Severe renal impairment. It will stain the teeth of children
under the age of 8 years — permanently. It is not used in this
age group for this reason.
Precautions:
Renal or hepatic impairment, those receiving drugs which may
damage the liver (oral contraceptives would be included here).
Long term treatment requires monitoring of kidney and liver
function and blood. This has consequences for those who
receive treatment for acne when many months of drug therapy
is given.
Effects:
Central nervous system: headaches, neck stiffness and pain,
vomiting and photophobia, benign intracranial hypertension
(especially children), ataxia, vertigo, dizziness.
Gastrointestinal: anorexia, nausea, vomiting, diarrhoea, irritation of mouth or tongue, black coat on tongue, sore throat,
burning sensation in the epigastrium, abdominal pain, liver
dysfunction, pancreatitis.
Urogenital: changes in renal function.
Skin: urticaria, photosensitivity, skin reddening.
Blood: anaemia, neutropenia, leucopenia, thrombocytopenia,
aplastic anaemia.
Allergic: swelling of the face, asthma, fever, painful swollen
joints, jaundice.

CHEM NAME	TRADE NAME	FORMULATION
chlor- tetracycline	AUREOMYCIN	250mg

1-2 four times daily.
Not for children.

	TRADE NAME	FORMULATION
	DETECLO	115.4mg with 115.4mg tetracycline 69.2mg demeclocycline

1 twice daily.
Not for children.

clomocycline	MEGACLOR	170mg

1-2 three or four times daily.
Not for children.

demeclocycline	LEDERMYCIN	150mg, 300mg

300mg twice daily.
Not for children.

doxycycline	NORDOX	100mg
	VIBRAMYCIN	100mg, 50mg/5ml

100mg daily.
Clearly stated as not for children. However the syrup form of
VIBRAMYCIN has dosages given for children of 2mg/Kg.

lymecycline	TETRALYSAL	408mg (= 300mg tetracycline)

1 twice daily.
Not for children.

minocycline	MINOCIN	100mg
	MINOCIN 50	50mg

100mg twice daily.
Not for children.

oxy- tetracycline	BERKMYCEN	250mg
	IMPERACIN	250mg
	OXYMYCIN	250mg
	TERRAMYCIN	250mg
	UNIMYCIN	250mg

250mg four times daily.
Clearly stated as not for children. However some formulations give a
children's dose as 25-50mg/Kg daily.

tetracycline	ACHROMYCIN	250mg, 125mg/5ml
	TETRACHEL	250mg

One four times daily.
Not for children.

	SUSTAMYCIN	250mg sustained-release

	TETRABID	250mg sustained-release

1 twice daily.
Not for children.

	MYSTECLIN	250mg with 250000 units nystatin 125mg/5ml with 25mg amphotericin

250-500mg four times daily.
Not for children.
With the addition of antifungal agents.

QUINOLONE

Commonly used for urinary tract infections including long-term prophylaxis.
Contraindications:
Children and young adults, liver disease, avoid excessive exposure to sunlight, epilepsy or history of epilepsy.
Effects:
General: tiredness, drowsiness, joint pain, restlessness.
Central nervous system: dizziness, headache, convulsions, vertigo, parasthesiae, benign intracranial hypertension (children and infants).
Psychological: confusion, psychosis, hallucinations, depression, confabulation, insomnia.
Gastrointestinal: nausea, diarrhoea, vomiting, epigastric and abdominal pain, gastric bleeding, changes in liver function.
Urogenital: changes in renal function.
Blood disorders: neutropenia, leucopenia, thrombocytopenia, pancytopenia, haemolytic anaemia.
Skin: skin rashes, itching, photosensitivity.
Special senses: visual disturbances such as blurred vision, lights appear bright, changes in colour perception.

CHEM NAME	TRADE NAME	FORMULATION
cinoxacin	CINOBAC	500mg

1 twice daily. Long term treatment — 1 at night.
Not for children.

ciprofloxacin	CIPROXIN	250mg

250-750mg twice daily.
Not for children.

enoxacin	COMPRECIN	200mg

1 twice daily for urinary tract infections. 2 twice daily for others.
Not for children.

nalidixic acid	NEGRAM	500mg, 300mg/5ml
	URIBEN	300mg/5ml

500mg-1G four times daily.
Children: under 3 months not recommended, 3 months-12 years up to 50mg/Kg daily.

	MICTRAL	660mg with sodium citrate, sodium bicarbonate, citric acid

One three times daily for three days.
Not for children.
Contains alkalising agents. These alkalinise urine in cases of urinary tract infection.

ofloxacin	TARIVID	200mg

1-4 usually for five to ten days.
Not for children.

MACROLIDE

Commonly used in infections of children.
Precautions:
Hepatic impairment, those receiving drugs which may damage the liver.
Effects:
Gastrointestinal: nausea, vomiting, diarrhoea, abdominal pain which in some cases may be severe, rectal irritation, changes in liver function, jaundice.
Diarrhoea may indicate the onset of a drug-induced colitis and so should be viewed with suspicion.
Allergy: anaphylaxis.
Skin: itching, nettle rash.
Special senses: hearing loss (reversible).

CHEM NAME	TRADE NAME	FORMULATION
erythromycin	ARPIMYCIN	125mg/5ml, 250mg/5ml, 500mg/5ml

1-2G daily.
Children: 30-100mg/Kg daily.

	ERYCEN	250mg, 500mg

	ERYMAX	250mg

1-2G daily.
Maintenance for acne 250mg once daily.
Not for children.

	ERYMAX SPRINKLE	125mg

Children: 30-50mg/Kg daily.

	ERYTHROCIN	250mg, 500mg
	ERYTHROMID	250mg
	ERYTHROMID DS	500mg
	RETCIN	250mg

1-2G daily.
Not for children.

	ERYTHROPED A	500mg, 1G sachets
	ERYTHROPED	250mg/5ml
	ERYTHROPED FORTE	500mg/5ml
	ERYTHROPED P.I.	125mg/5ml
	ERYTHROPED SUGAR-FREE	250mg

1-2G daily.
Children: under 2 years 250mg, 2-8 years 500mg, over 8 years 1G. All
twice daily.

	ILOSONE	250mg, 500mg, 125mg/5ml, 250mg/5ml

250mg four times daily. Maximum 4G daily.
Children: 20-50mg/Kg daily.

FUSIDIC ACID

Precautions:
Liver function should be monitored in long-term therapy.
Special care should be exercised in those with pre-existing liver
problems or if high doses are given.
Effects:
Gastrointestinal: jaundice particularly in young and elderly.

CHEM NAME	TRADE NAME	FORMULATION
sodium fusidate	FUCIDIN	250mg, 250mg/5ml

15ml or 500mg three times daily.
Children: under 1 year 1ml/Kg daily. At ages 1-5 years 5ml, 5-12 years
10ml. Both three times daily.

SULPHONAMIDE

Not so often seen nowadays since the advent of newer antibiotics with fewer side-effects. Its main presentation is in conjunction with folic acid inhibitors (see SEPTRIN etc).

Precautions:
Severe reactions such as Stevens-Johnson syndrome and blood disorders of serious types may occur.
Caution in kidney and liver disease, dehydration and blood disorders.

Effects:
General: fever, drowsiness.
Cardiovascular: cyanosis.
Central nervous system: headache, neuritis.
Psychological: depression, lack of concentration.
Gastrointestinal: nausea, vomiting, anorexia, pancreatitis.
Urogenital: haematuria, anuria, crystalluria.
Endocrine: hypoglycaemia.
Skin: rashes.
Blood: haemolytic anaemia, leucopenia.
Special senses: optic neuritis.
Allergic: respiratory reactions including cough and breathlessness, nephritis, hepatitis, agranulocytosis, thrombocytopenia, pancytopenia.

CHEM NAME	TRADE NAME	FORMULATION
sulfameto- pyrazine 2G once weekly. Not for children.	KELFIZINE W	2G
sulphacarbamide	UROMIDE	500mg with 50mg phenazopyridine
2 three times daily. Children: half-1 three times daily. This contains an anaesthetic agent which is added to help relieve the pain of urinary tract infections.		

FOLIC ACID INHIBITOR

These drugs are given either alone or mixed with a sulphonamide antibiotic. They are commonly used for bacterial infections of the respiratory and urinary tract.

Contraindications:
Renal impairment where blood levels cannot be monitored regularly, anaemia due to Vitamin B12 or folic acid deficiency.
Precautions:
Renal impairment. Regular blood checks should be performed during long-term therapy.
Effects:
Central nervous system: headache.
Gastrointestinal: nausea, vomiting, glossitis, colitis.
Blood disorders: anaemia, leucopenia, thrombocytopenia, aplastic anaemia, pancytopenia.
Skin: rash, itching.

CHEM NAME	TRADE NAME	FORMULATION
trimethoprim	IPRAL	100mg, 200mg
	MONOTRIM	100mg, 200mg
	SYRAPRIM	100mg, 300mg
	TIEMPE	100mg, 200mg
TRIMOGAL		100mg, 200mg
	TRIMOPAN	100mg, 200mg

200mg twice daily.

	IPRAL PAED.	50mg/5ml
	MONOTRIM SUSP.	50mg/5ml
	TRIMOPAN SUSP.	50mg/5ml

Children: under 2 months not recommended, 2-6 months 2.5ml, 6 months-6 years 5ml, 6-12 years 10ml. All twice daily.

	BACTRIM	80mg with 400mg sulphamethoxazole and /5ml
	COMOX	80mg with 400mg sulphamethoxazole
	FECTRIM STANDARD	80mg with 400mg sulpha-methoxazole
	LARATRIM SUSP.	80mg with 400mg sulphamethoxazole/5ml
	SEPTRIN	80mg with 400mg sulphamethoxazole and /5ml

1-3 tabs. or 5-15ml twice daily.
Children: 6-12 years 1 tab. or 5ml twice daily.

	BACTRIM DOUBLE STRENGTH	160mg with 800mg sulphamethoxazole
	COMOX FORTE	160mg with 800mg sulphamethoxazole
	FECTRIM FORTE	160mg with 800mg

	sulphamethoxazole
LARATRIM FORTE	160mg with 800mg sulphamethoxazole
SEPTRIN FORTE	160mg with 800mg sulphamethoxazole

Half to one and a half twice daily
Not for children.

BACTRIM PAED. SYRUP	40mg with 200mg sulphamethoxazole/5ml
CHEMOTRIM Paed.	40mg with 200mg sulphamethoxazole/5ml
COMOX PAED. SYRUP	40mg with 200mg sulphamethoxazole/5ml
LARATRIM PAED. SUSP.	40mg with 200mg sulphamethoxazole/5ml
SEPTRIN PAED. SUSP.	40mg with 200mg sulphamethoxazole/5ml

Children: 6 weeks-5 months 2.5ml, 6 months-5 years 5ml, 6-12 years 10ml. All twice daily.

BACTRIM PAED. TABS.	20mg with 100mg sulphamethoxazole
FECTRIM PAED.	20mg with 100mg sulphamethoxazole
SEPTRIN PAED. TABS.	20mg with 100mg sulphamethoxazole

Children: 2-5 years 2 twice daily, 6-12 years 4 twice daily.
These also contain a sulphonamide (see above).

ANTIBACTERIAL

This particular drug is used in cases of urinary tract infections.
Contraindications:
Not for use in dehydration, hepatic impairment, severe renal impairment.
Effects:
Gastrointestinal: nausea, vomiting, indigestion.
Urogenital: bladder irritation.
Skin: rashes.

CHEM NAME	TRADE NAME	FORMULATION
hexamine	HIPREX	1G

1G twice daily.
Children: Not under 6 years, 6-12 years half adult dose.

NITROIMIDAZOLE

These are very powerful drugs. They frequently make people feel quite ill. They are used for protozoal infections such as trichomoniasis and giardiasis.

Precautions:

Patients should avoid alcohol during treatment.

Clinical and laboratory monitoring should be performed if treatment is longer than 10 days.

Effects:

General: drowsiness, intolerance to alcohol (in 25%).

Central nervous system: dizziness, headache, ataxia, convulsions, peripheral neuropathy.

Psychological: depression.

Gastrointestinal: metallic taste in mouth, furred tongue, nausea, vomiting, abdominal pains, diarrhoea.

Urogenital: darkening of urine, discomfort on urination.

Allergy: angioedema, anaphylaxis.

Blood disorders: leucopenia, neutropenia.

Skin: rashes, pruritus.

CHEM NAME	TRADE NAME	FORMULATION
metronidazole	FLAGYL	200mg, 400mg, 200mg/5ml
	METROLYL	200mg, 400mg
	NIDAZOL	200mg
	ZADSTAT	200mg
400mg three times daily.		
Children: 7.5mg/Kg three times daily.		
tinidazole	FASIGYN	500mg
2 daily.		
This may also cause vertigo.		

ANTIFUNGAL AGENTS

These are commonly used for fungal infections of the skin and mucous membranes. Conditions such as vaginal candidiasis ('thrush') are invariably treated by such agents. Patients often enter a vicious circle of vaginal discharge, antifungal agent, disappearance of discharge, reappearance of discharge, antifungal agent and so on. It is essential to remember that fungi are opportunist pathogens — that is they are very commonly present in many people and only become a problem when resistance is lowered as in antibiotic or oral contraceptive use. General treatment is essential as well as considering possible allergic components to the condition.

POLYENE ANTIBIOTICS
Effects:
Gastrointestinal: nausea, vomiting, diarrhoea.

CHEM NAME	TRADE NAME	FORMULATION
amphotericin	FUNGILIN	100mg, 100mg/ml

100-200mg four times daily.
Children: 1ml four times daily.

nystatin	NYSTAN	500000 units, 100000 units/ml

1ml for oral infections and 5ml or 1-2 tablets for intestinal infections. Both four times daily.
Children: 1ml four times daily.

TRIAZOLE
Precautions:
Liver function tests may be affected. If so there may be a flareup of Hepatitis B (serum hepatitis) in those with a history of this illness.
Effects:
Central nervous system: headache.
Gastrointestinal: nausea, abdominal discomfort.

CHEM NAME	TRADE NAME	FORMULATION
fluconazole	DIFLUCAN	50mg, 200mg

50mg daily. For systemic infection 200-400mg once daily.
Not for children.

itraconazole	SPORANOX	100mg

1 daily for most infections.
Not for children or elderly.

GRISEOFULVIN
Contraindications:
Porphyria, severe liver disease, systemic lupus erythematosus.

Precautions:
Avoid sunlight.
Effects:
General: drowsiness, tiredness.
Central nervous system: headache (in 50% and may be severe), dizziness.
Psychological: confusion, depression, irritability, insomnia. These are all made worse by the concurrent use of alcohol.
Gastrointestinal: gastric discomfort, feeling of fullness in stomach, anorexia, nausea, diarrhoea, black furry tongue, angular stomatitis, disturbance of taste.
Skin: rashes, urticaria, photosensitivity.
Blood: leucopenia, neutropenia, monocytosis.
Special senses: visual disturbances.

CHEM NAME	TRADE NAME	FORMULATION
griseofulvin	FULCIN	125mg, 500mg
	GRISOVIN	125mg, 500mg

500mg-1G daily.
Children: 10mg/Kg daily.

IMIDAZOLE

Mild gastrointestinal effects are seen with DAKTARIN which is administered orally.
Local application may produce a contact dermatitis with itching, redness and soreness.
Example – ketoconazole
Contraindications:
Liver disease.
Precautions:
Hepatitis may occur so liver function must be checked prior to long term treatment. Fatalities have occurred.
Effects:
General: drowsiness.
Central nervous system: headache, dizziness.
Gastrointestinal: nausea, vomiting, indigestion, constipation, changes in liver function, hepatitis.
Psychological: anxiety.
Endocrine: gynaecomastia.
Skin: itching, urticaria.

CHEM NAME	TRADE NAME	FORMULATION
clotrimazole	CANESTEN	cream, vaginal tablets

Used in the treatment of fungal infections of skin and vagina.

econazole	ECONACORT	With hydrocortisone 1% – with addition of mild corticosteroid
	ECOSTATIN	1% cream/lotion/spray/powder
	GYNO-PEVARYL	pessaries
	PEVARYL	1% cream/lotion/powder
	PEVARYL TC	1% with triamcinolone 0.1% (cream) With the addition of a potent corticosteroid

These are all local applications and are used for a wide variety of fungal disorders of skin, vagina, nails and so on.

ketoconazole	NIZORAL	200mg, 100mg/5ml

200-400mg daily.
Children: 3mg/Kg daily.

miconazole	DAKTARIN	250mg, oral gel 25mg/ml

1 tab. four times daily or 5-10mg gel four times daily.
Children: under 2 years 2.5ml twice daily, 2-6 years 5ml twice daily, over 6 years 5ml four times daily.

	GYNO-DAKTARIN	cream, pessary

Used in vaginal fungal infections.

ANTIVIRAL AGENTS

In recent years there have been some developments in substances available to combat viral disease. These have always been difficult to treat by conventional medicine because viral activity tends to be intracellular. Therefore any treatment aimed at damaging the virus will usually damage the cell. However there are some limited treatments used against herpes infections such as herpes simplex and zoster as well as HIV (human immunovirus) infection.

ACYCLOVIR

This is used in the treatment of severe recurrent herpes simplex of the genitalia and other sites.

It is also used in the treatment of herpes zoster and although it may reduce the pain of the attack there is no evidence that it alters the incidence of post-herpetic neuralgia.

Effects:

General: fatigue.

Central nervous system: headaches, mild neurological reactions.

Gastrointestinal: nausea, vomiting, diarrhoea, abdominal pain, changes in liver function.

Urogenital: changes in renal function.

Skin: rashes

CHEM NAME	TRADE NAME	FORMULATION
acyclovir	ZOVIRAX	200mg, 400mg, 800mg, 200mg/5ml, 5% cream

AMANTADINE

This drug is also used in the treatment of Parkinson's disease. In its role as an anti-viral agent it is used to protect against the development of or to treat influenza and herpes zoster.

See Chapter 10 for details of effects.

CHEM NAME	TRADE NAME	FORMULATION
amantadine	MANTADINE	100mg
	SYMMETREL	100mg, 50mg/5ml

Influenza treatment: 1 twice daily for 5-7 days.

Influenza prevention: 1 twice daily for 7-10 days.

Herpes zoster: 1 twice daily for 7-10 days.

Children: not under 10 years. Over 10 years only for prevention or treatment of influenza: 1 daily.

IDOXURIDINE

This is used to treat herpes simplex and herpes zoster. Local applications are used several times each day.

Contraindications:

This drug definitely causes foetal deformities in animal experimentation. Therefore this must never be given to pregnant women or those who may become pregnant. All drugs must be used in pregnancy only in an emergency.

It must not be used in those with dermatographia. This is a condition of presumed allergic origin where scraping the skin produces a characteristic appearance of redness and swelling. So much so that is it possible for letters and words to show up after light scratching.

Effects:

Gastrointestinal: taste in the mouth.

Skin: stinging at the site of use.

CHEM NAME	TRADE NAME	FORMULATION
idoxuridine	HERPID	5%
	IDURIDIN	5%
	VIRUDOX	5%

Local application for herpes simplex and herpes zoster.

INOSINE

This is used to treat herpes simplex infections and genital warts (in conjunction with treatment to burn them away).

Precautions:

Uric acid is the end product of inosine metabolism and so care must be exercised in those with impaired renal function or gout.

Effects:

Blood: raised levels of uric acid.

CHEM NAME	TRADE NAME	FORMULATION
inosine	IMMUNOVIR	500mg

4G daily for 1-2 weeks.

ZIDOVUDINE (also known as AZT)

Although this is classed as an anti-viral drug it has more in common with chemotherapeutic agents used in the treatment of cancer. It was originally developed in 1964 for just this use. It was only in 1987 that it was licenced for use in AIDS and AIDS-related conditions. More recently it has been advocated for use in HIV positive patients to reputedly slow the development of AIDS.

This whole subject has occupied many books on its own. I would say here that the conventional treatment of disease such as cancer and AIDS has very toxic effects. The emphasis is on the symptoms and the tumours. The patient is very much relegated to a subsidiary position. Alternative medicine has a very different approach and there are many examples of non-toxic cancer therapies with proven high success rates. My own approach to such patients is to use a combination of treatments – acupuncture and Chinese herbs, daily visualisation, dietary changes – as well as perhaps healing, massage and so on. This multiple approach is essential to offer patients as much help as possible.

The assumption that HIV definitely leads to AIDS in all cases and that AIDS has a 100% mortality is clearly not true and the people with the longest survival rates in the highest state of health are those who have declined AZT medication and sought other methods.

The pressure by the medical profession and pharmaceutical industry on patients to take this drug is quite scandalous. There is little open discussion about its risks and the original trials conducted in the USA were not conducted on a satisfactory double-blind basis. Patients had the tablets analysed to see if they were taking AZT or merely placebo. Many of those on placebo either obtained AZT themselves or shared with others on the trial.

Treatments for serious life-threatening illness such as cancer and AIDS would be included in category V on page 20. Therefore help from a conventionally trained practitioner may be advisable.

As with conventional treatment of many disorders some patients feel better at the beginning. They have more energy and white cells increase in number. After 3–6 months however the white cell count stabilises and then starts to fall. After 12 months the patient is usually worse off in terms of their numbers of white cells and general health.

Contraindications:
Not to be given to those with a haemoglobin below 7.5G% or a neutrophil count below 0.75x109. It is toxic to bone marrow and causes resultant problems in 30%. These will require blood transfusions at monthly intervals.

Precautions:
The white cell count is further diminished if analgesics such as paracetamol are taken long term.

Effects:
General: malaise, tiredness, fever, myalgia, sweat.ng, generalised pain, chills, influenza-like symptoms, muscle weakness.
Cardiovascular: chest pain.
Respiratory: cough, dyspnoea.
Central nervous system: intolerable headache, paraesthesia, dizziness, convulsions (described in one patient), encephalitis.
Psychological: insomnia, anxiety, mental dullness, depression, confusion (described in one patient).
Gastrointestinal: nausea, vomiting, anorexia, abdominal pain, diarrhoea, indigestion, flatulence, unpleasant taste in mouth.
Urogenital: frequency of urination, impotence.
Blood: anaemia, neutropenia, leucopenia.
This occurs more frequently in those with AIDS than with ARC, with low Vitamin B12 levels or if paracetamol is taken.
Skin: rash, urticaria, itching.

CHEM NAME	TRADE NAME	FORMULATION
zidovudine	RETROVIR	100mg, 250mg

200-300mg or 3.5mg/Kg every four hours.
Not for children.

5 TRICKY CASES

Drugs Necessary For Life

This is one extreme of drug use but is not as common as one would first suppose. If patients do take these I would suggest seeking the help of a sympathetic doctor.

These are Category V drugs.

CARDIAC DRUGS

The drugs I am thinking of here are those given for severe and serious arrhythmias often arising from the ventricle. They are not commonly seen.

CHEM NAME	TRADE NAME	FORMULATION
amiodarone	CORDARONE-X	
disopyramide	DIRYTHMIN SA	
	RYTHMODAN	
flecainide	TAMBOCOR	
isoprenaline	SAVENTRINE	
mexiletine	MEXITIL	
procainamide	PROCAINAMIDE DURULES	
	PRONESTYL	
propafenone	ARYTHMOL	
quinidine	KIDITARD	
	KINIDIN DURULES	
tocainide	TONOCARD	
verapamil	BERKATENS	
	CORDILOX	
	SECURON	

These should not be touched without liason with a convention-ally trained practitioner as any inappropriate reduction in dosage may lead to a fatal cardiac arrhythmia.

A note here about betablockers. These may be given on occasion to prevent or treat cardiac arrhythmias so check their indication in each case. The type of arrhythmia they will be given for are those of atrial origin leading to palpitations. These are not as severe as those of ventricular origin. Betablockers can be dealt with in most instances as outlined in Chapter 7. Take care if there is severe underlying structural heart disease.

Hormone Deficiency States

Here I am talking about hormones given because of underactivity of an endocrine gland due to a pathological process. It does not include oestrogen given to women during or after the menopause, the contraceptive pill or progestogens used for infertility, premenstrual syndrome and so on.

Diabetes Mellitus

First, a differentiation must be made between insulin dependent and non-insulin dependent types. The problem for the patient and the practitioner is that diabetes mellitus treated by either insulin or hypoglycaemic agents may be complicated by the development of hypoglycaemia — 'hypos'. This may manifest as merely hunger or lightheadedness or may develop into coma. Death can occur if the blood sugar level falls severely.

In treating patients the risk of such a state developing should be minimised as much as possible. In the case of patients who take insulin, this acts rapidly, the dosage and adjustment of dosage is complex and so monitoring is important. It is better if such cases are supervised by a doctor. During treatment the blood sugar should be monitored frequently every day. Once treatment is instituted the blood sugar is likely to fall. Insulin dosage needs to be adjusted in response to this. This will be a continuous process as, hopefully, the condition improves.

It is unusual for people to be able to stop their insulin completely but either the dose can be reduced or cases of 'brittle' or unstable diabetes become stable. In both cases the patient feels better in themselves with more energy.

In non-insulin dependent diabetes mellitus most cases are relatively simple to manage. Again, the problem with the hypoglycaemic agents is that they can induce hypoglycaemia. With due care it is possible to begin a strict diet and stop the drugs whilst treating. Monitoring of the blood sugar will ensure that very high levels are not attained. The patient should also take steps to ensure that their activities do not lead to raised blood sugar such as stressful situations, smoking, the taking of coffee or stimulant drugs.

As treatment progresses the blood sugar level should fall as the patient's condition improves. Do not worry if the patient only feels better initially with improved energy levels but little change in the blood sugar. Falls in sugar level follow these improvements.

Symptoms and signs to be concerned about in either type of diabetes are a rising blood sugar level, deterioration in feeling of wellness, the appearance of ketones in the urine and worsening of symptoms such as frequency and volume of urination, thirst and appetite, occurrence of hypoglycaemic episodes.

In these cases either more frequent treatment is necessary, a review of treatment required or conventional medical treatment may need to be instituted in extreme situations.

HYPOGLYCAEMIC AGENTS

These drugs are used in the treatment of non-insulin dependent diabetes (variously known as maturity onset or late onset). They stimulate the pancreas to produce more insulin. They do nothing to remedy the underlying problem which is one of inadequate output of insulin to meet the needs of the body — commonly due to inappropriate diet, emotional stresses and strains or the effects of long standing imbalances.

SULPHONYLUREA

Contraindications:
Insulin-dependent diabetes mellitus, serious impairment of kidney, liver or adrenal cortex or situations of unusual stress such as surgical operations or pregnancy.

Certain drugs alter the hypoglycaemic effect including some antibiotics, salicylates (aspirin-like compounds), corticosteroids, oral contraceptives, diuretics and excessive laxative use.

Effects:
Gastrointestinal: mild gastrointestinal upsets. Changes in liver function.
Endocrine: hypoglycaemia.
Blood disorders: leucopenia, thrombocytopenia.
Skin: rashes.

CHEM NAME	TRADE NAME	FORMULATION
acetohexamide 250mg–1.5G daily	DIMELOR	500mg
chlorpropamide 100–250mg daily. Maximum 500mg daily.	DIABINESE	100mg, 250mg
glibenclamide	CALABREN	5mg

	DAONIL	5mg
	EUGLUCON	2.5mg, 5mg
	LIBANIL	2.5mg
	MALIX	2.5mg
	SEMI-DAONIL	2.5mg

5mg daily. Maximum 15mg daily.

| glicazide | DIAMICRON | 80mg |

40–80mg daily. Maximum 320mg daily.

| glipizide | GLIBENESE | 5mg |
| | MINODIAB | 2.5mg, 5mg |

Maintenance 2.5–30mg daily. Maximum 40mg daily.

| gliquidone | GLURENORM | 30mg |

45–60mg. Maximum 180mg daily.

| tolazamide | TOLANASE | 100mg, 250mg |

100–250mg daily. Maximum 1G daily.

| tolbutamide | RASTINON | 500mg |

Maintenance 1–3 daily.

BULKING AGENT

These may be used together with a hypoglycaemic agent. High residue (fibre) diets have a similar effect in lowering blood sugar.
Contraindications:
Oesophageal disease or intestinal obstruction.
Precautions:
Hypoglycaemia may occur at the beginning of treatment.
Effects:
Gastrointestinal: flatulence, changes in bowel habit, nausea.

CHEM NAME	TRADE NAME	FORMULATION
guar gum	GUAREM	5G sachets
	GUARINA	5G sachets

Maximum of 3 daily.

BIGUANIDE
Contraindications:
Chronic liver disease, cardiac failure, recent myocardial infarction and alcoholism.

Precautions:
Regular monitoring of renal function should be carried out as well as an annual estimation of Vitamin B12 levels.
Effects:
Gastrointestinal: nausea, vomiting, diarrhoea.
Endocrine: development of lactic acidosis. This is a potentially fatal condition which may occur with diabetic patients where there are metabolic disturbances as a result of the build-up of lactic acid in the tissues. The condition is a medical emergency and requires in-patient treatment.

CHEM NAME	TRADE NAME	FORMULATION
metformin	GLUCOPHAGE	500mg, 850mg
	ORABET	500mg, 850mg

Maintenance usually 2x850mg or 3x500mg daily. Maximum of 3G daily.

Thyroid Disease

THYROXINE

CHEM NAME	TRADE NAME	FORMULATION
liothyronine	TERTROXIN	20mcg
80–100mcg daily.		
thyroxine	ELTROXIN	50mcg, 100mcg
50–100mcg daily. Maximum 150–300mcg daily.		

Thyroid replacement therapy is used in cases of hypothyroidism — underactivity of thyroid gland function. The disease tends to be variable in its manifestations and there may be a progressive element. Annual checks of thyroid hormone levels are advised conventionally.
When treating such patients thyroid function may improve so that the dose of thyroid hormone is then too much. When treating such patients I arrange for blood levels to be checked every 3 or 6 months with reversion to annual checks after treatment has ended. If necessary the dosage of thyroid replacement is altered in accordance with the level in the blood.

CASE

Man aged 73 years came for treatment because of general tiredness, listlessness and a tendency in recent months to catch colds and upper respiratory tract infections.

He had a heart attack several years ago and since then had been taking INDERAL. Diagnosed as having underactive thyroid 10 or so years ago.

His symptoms included sore throat and dry cough since a heavy cold when he was given antibiotics. He had general debility, wheezy chest and a loss of appetite.

Medication:

> INDERAL 40mg three times daily.
> thyroxine 0.1mg three times daily.

Apart from his general condition several comments can be made with relation to his drugs.

INDERAL, a betablocker, is sedative in its action and so leads to tiredness, debility, cold extremities. It can cause wheezing. It was taken in this case to prevent a second heart attack.

A study performed in Scandinavia some years ago seemed to show that giving betablockers after a heart attack could prevent a further attack. There has been some doubt cast on this by subsequent work.

This dose of thyroxine is larger than usually required. He had not had a blood check by his GP for at least 5 years.

Whilst treatment began for his presenting problem it was important to get a thyroxine check. The result was 207nmol/l (normal range is 70–150nmol/l).

The thyroxine supplementation was reduced to 0.1mg twice daily.

After several weeks treatment it was time to work on the INDERAL which was no longer necessary. The point with betablockers is to ensure slow reduction to prevent the possibility of myocardial infarction (see Chapter 7). In this case it was possible to reduce the drug by 40mg every 2 weeks. After 6 weeks he had stopped it. In cases of hypertension or angina it will clearly take longer because of the underlying disease.

A further thyroxine estimation performed after 3 months revealed a level of 128nmol/l which is normal. Treatment continued and a blood check 6 months later showed a level of 180nmol/l. This necessitated a reduction to 0.1mg daily alternating with 0.1mg twice daily. A blood test after 3 months showed the level had dropped to 131nmol/l.

This reveals the importance of regular monitoring and how thyroid function can recover with constitutional treatment.

ANTI-THYROID DRUGS

These are used in the treatment of thyrotoxicosis. When dealing with patients who take such medication you need to bear in mind that this can be a serious condition. Management must include estimation of serum thyroxine levels.

Most patients tend to decide on conventional treatment when first diagnosed and so present for alternative treatment at a later date. Improvement as a result of alternative treatment will be observed in the clinical condition as well as serum thyroxine levels. Reduction of the carbimazole can take place as levels fall.

Conventional management is for the patient to take the drug for a year or so. Effective alternative treatment may well reduce this period and end in an improved state of health. As with many conditions it is clearly more beneficial if patients present for treatment as soon as they notice symptoms (if not before). Delay, as is often the case when conventional investigations are undertaken, will make it more difficult to treat such patients.
Precautions:
This drug can damage the bone marrow and so all patients must be told to report symptoms such as sore throats, mouth ulcers, bruising or those of anaemia.
Effects:
Central nervous system: headache.
Gastrointestinal: nausea, gastric upset.
Blood: agranulocytosis.
Skin: itching, rashes, hair loss.

CHEM NAME	TRADE NAME	FORMULATION
carbimazole	NEO-MERCAZOLE	5mg, 20mg
Maintenance of 5–15mg daily for 6–18 months.		

Diabetes Insipidus

This is a rare condition due to either pituitary or renal disease where there is insufficiency of or failure to respond to antidiuretic hormone.

CHEM NAME	TRADE NAME	FORMULATION
antidiuretic hormone	PITRESSIN	injection
desmopressin	DDAVP	intranasal spray
	DESMOSPRAY	intranasal spray
lypressin	SYNTOPRESSIN	nasal spray

Desmopressin is also used in the treatment of enuresis in children and adults. It must never be given to children under the age of 5 years. Every 3 months there must be an assessment by stopping the drug for at least one week. The use of such a drug seems to be a very powerful way of trying to prevent a symptom which is usually very amenable to treatment by other means.

Addison's Disease
(Insufficiency of Adrenal Cortex)

Such patients take a mixture of corticosteroids of two types, a glucocorticoid such as cortisone or prednisolone (see Chapter 12) and a mineralocorticoid. These drugs must not be altered or stopped at all without monitoring which must be performed in conjunction with conventional medical advice.

Do not confuse the use of these drugs here and when given for their anti-inflammatory effect in disorders such as rheumatoid arthritis, ulcerative colitis, asthma and so on. Cortisone and hydrocortisone have mixed glucocorticoid/mineralocorticoid actions and so may be prescribed in inflammatory disease. Fludrocortisone is only ever seen in cases of insufficiency of the adrenal cortex.

MINERALOCORTICOIDS

CHEM NAME	TRADE NAME	FORMULATION
cortisone	CORTELAN	25mg
	CORTISTAB	5mg, 25mg
	CORTISYL	25mg
25–40mg daily		
fludrocortisone	FLORINEF	0.1mg
0.05–0.3mg daily		
hydrocortisone	HYDROCORTISTAB	20mg
	HYDROCORTONE	10mg, 20mg
10–30mg daily.		

6 PSYCHOACTIVE DRUGS

These are used in the treatment of the various standard classifications of psychological disease. They are also given for a wide range of other disorders which are categorised as 'neurotic' in origin or in diseases which occur in patients who exhibit 'neurotic' symptoms.

Antidepressants

These usually are included in Category II (Chapter 3). The exceptions are those circumstances where weak patients take large doses for long periods of time. Withdrawal in these cases may lead to severe reactions. They must then be considered as Category III drugs.

There are several groups of drugs available. The commonest ones used are the tricyclic antidepressants and the monoamine oxidase inhibitors. They have been in common use since the early 1960's.

As is evidenced by their chemical names most are very closely related and are good examples of 'me-too' drugs[6]. There is little to choose between them in terms of safety and occurrence of side-effects. They all have a degree of sedative action although some are combined with tranquillisers if there is anxiety with the depression.

They are given in the day or commonly at night because of the associated sedation.

Depression, in common with many psychological disorders, is thought conventionally to be due to problems with transmitter substances in the central nervous system. Antidepressants aim to change these levels.

It can be seen from the list of effects that antidepressants heat the body up and have similar effects to amphetamines ('speed'). They are 'uppers' and are effective in lifting the black mood of depression. However, because depression is usually only the surface feeling and there is invariably an underlying emotion the drugs may only serve to give an improvement on a superficial level. They make no attempt at resolving or treating the underlying process, indeed this is now more likely to be ignored because the patient feels subjectively improved. The continual effect of drug dosage will be one of damage to organs both structurally and energetically.

TRICYCLIC GROUP

Category II in most cases.
Category III if large doses are taken for a long time in weak patients where the release of a suppression would be difficult to deal with.

Contraindications:
They should not be used with the monoamine oxidase inhibitor group of antidepressants.

Because of their effect on the heart (see effects) they should not be given to people who are recovering from a coronary thrombosis or those who suffer from irregular heart rhythms (this would include palpitations).

Not to be used in mania because they may cause manic states or delusional conditions.

They should not be given to those with severe liver disease or children under the age of 6 years — this has implications for children with enuresis (bedwetting) — see TOFRANIL (imipramine).

Precautions:
History of epilepsy, evidence of impaired liver function, history of urinary retention, prostatic hypertrophy, narrow-angle glaucoma or just increased intra-ocular pressure, cardiovascular disorders, hyperthyroid patients, those taking thyroid medication or anticholinergic agents.

The elderly are especially liable to effects concerning the cardiovascular and central nervous systems.

When this group of drugs is used for depression in schizophrenia the psychosis worsens.

Behavioural changes can be seen in children receiving treatment for nocturnal enuresis. Tricyclic antidepressant overdosage is the commonest cause of accidental death in children under 5 in the UK.

Effects:
This is quite a list and shows the power of these agents. They can cause many problems in many areas of the body.

General: weakness, sedation, fatigue, oedema of face and tongue, weight gain.

Cardiovascular: hypotension, postural hypotension, hypertension, rapid heart rate, palpitations.

Central nervous system: headache, parasthesiae such as numbness and tingling in the extremities, incoordination, ataxia, dysarthria, tremors, convulsions, Parkinsonian symptoms of tremor, rigidity and slow movement, tinnitus, dizziness, peripheral neuropathy, stroke, EEG changes.

Gastrointestinal: dry mouth, nausea, indigestion, vomiting, decreased or increased appetite, weight gain or loss, stomatitis, unpleasant taste, diarrhoea, constipation, parotid swelling, black tongue, paralytic ileus, changes in liver function, jaundice, hepatitis.

Psychological: confusional states, disturbed concentration and memory, disorientation, delusions, hallucinations, hypomania (in about 10%), excitement, anxiety, restlessness, insomnia, nightmares, drowsiness.

Aggressiveness may be seen with imipramine and amitryptiline.

Endocrine: testicular swelling, gynaecomastia, breast enlargement, milk secretion from the breast.

Urogenital: urinary retention, urinary frequency, impotence, increased or decreased libido, delayed ejaculation, painful ejaculation.

Skin: rashes, nettle rash, photosensitisation, alopecia, sweating, purpura.

Blood disorders: leucopenia, eosinophilia, thrombocytopenia.

Agranulocytosis leading to deaths has occurred. Blood counts should be performed in those who develop fever, sore throat or other signs of infection during course of medication.

Special senses: blurred vision.

CHEM NAME	TRADE NAME	FORMULATION
amitryptiline	DOMICAL	10mg, 25mg, 50mg.
	ELAVIL	10mg, 25mg.
	TRYPTIZOL	10mg, 25mg, 50mg.

Usual maintenance, 50-100mg at night. Maximum 200mg daily.
Elderly, initially 10-50mg daily.

	LENTIZOL	25mg, 50mg sustained-release

50mg at night. Maximum 100mg daily.
Elderly: initially 25-75 mg daily.

	LIMBITROL 5	12.5mg with 5mg chlordiazepoxide.
	LIMBITROL 10	25mg with 10mg chlordiazepoxide.

One three times daily for depression with anxiety. The larger doses are used for more severe cases.
Not for the elderly.
With the addition of a benzodiazepine tranquilliser.

	TRIPTAFEN	25mg with 2mg perphenazine.

TRIPTAFEN-M   10mg with 2mg
perphenazine.
One three times daily with one at night if necessary for depression
with anxiety. To be reassessed by the prescriber after three months.
With the addition of a phenothiazine tranquilliser.

amoxapine   ASENDIS   25mg,50mg,100mg, 150mg
150-250mg daily. Maximum 300mg daily.
Elderly: maximum 150mg daily.
This seems to cause more neurological problems than others.

butryptiline   EVADYNE   25mg, 50mg.
Maintenance, 25mg three times daily. Maximum of 100-150mg daily.

clomipramine   ANAFRANIL   10mg, 25mg, 50mg,
25mg/ml.
     ANAFRANIL SR   75mg sustained-release
30-150mg daily.
Elderly: initially 10mg daily. Maximum 75mg daily.
This drug may prevent ejaculation completely.

desipramine   PERTOFRAN   25mg.
2 three or four times daily.
Elderly, initially one daily.

dothiepin   PROTHIADEN   25mg, 75mg.
75-150mg daily.

doxepin   SINEQUAN   10mg, 25mg, 50mg, 75mg.
10-100mg three times daily, or up to 100mg as a single dose at night.

fluoxetine   PROZAC   20mg
1 daily. Maximum 4 daily.
Elderly: 1 daily. Maximum 3 daily.

imipramine   TOFRANIL   10mg, 25mg.
50mg three or four times daily.
Elderly 10-25mg three times daily.
This drug is also used for nocturnal enuresis when it is given in
syrup form. It seems to be a very drastic and potentially harmful
treatment for such a condition.

iprindole   PRONDOL   15mg, 30mg.
15-30mg three times daily. Maximum 60mg three times daily.
Elderly, initially 15mg three times daily.
Jaundice occurs more commonly with this drug. It is due to stasis of
bile within the liver and is allergic in origin.

lofepramine   GAMANIL   70mg.
1 morning and 1-2 at night.
Tremor is more marked with this drug.

nortryptiline   ALLEGRON   10mg, 25mg.
     AVENTYL   10mg, 25mg.
Maintenance usually 30-75mg daily.

Elderly: initially 10mg three times daily.

	MOTIPRESS	30mg with 1.5mg fluphenazine.
	MOTIVAL	10mg with 0.5mg fluphenazine.

Dosage is one daily at night of MOTIPRESS and one two or three times daily of MOTIVAL for a maximum of three months.
With the addition of a phenothiazine tranquilliser.

protryptiline   CONCORDIN   5mg, 10mg.
15-60mg daily.
Elderly, initially 5mg three times daily.

trimipramine   SURMONTIL   10mg, 25mg, 50mg.
50-75mg daily.
Elderly, initially 10-25mg three times daily.

MONOAMINE OXIDASE INHIBITORS (MAOI)

Category II in most cases.
Category III if large doses are taken for a long time in a weak patient where the release of a suppression may cause great difficulties for the patient.

Contraindications:
History of liver damage or insufficiency (since they can cause toxic hepatitis) and those with cerebrovascular disease.
They should not be given within 14 days of taking tricyclic antidepressants.

Special precautions:
MAOI increase the effects of drugs such as opiates, adrenaline, amphetamines and other sympathomimetic amines, dopamine, and levodopa, as well as anti-hypertensives, hypoglycaemic agents, anti-Parkinson drugs, local anaesthetics and central nervous system depressants such as alcohol.
It should be withdrawn 2 weeks before surgery or dentistry.
Patients should avoid cheese, foods containing high proportion of degraded protein such as Oxo, Bovril, Marmite etc during treatment and up to 14 days after ceasing treatment.
Patients should be told to restrict alcohol intake, to avoid heavy red wines and warned about self-medication especially with cold cures. Great caution must be exercised in the elderly or agitated, those with evidence of cardiovascular disease, epilepsy, blood disorders, phaeochromocytoma, patients with liver toxicity, or diabetes mellitus.

Effects:
General: drowsiness, weakness, fatigue.
Cardiovascular: palpitations, postural hypotension, oedema (diuretics have no effect).
Gastrointestinal: increased appetite and weight, nausea, vomiting, dry mouth, constipation.
Central nervous system: dizziness, headache, parasthesiae, peripheral neuritis, muscle tremor, convulsions, EEG changes.
Psychological: insomnia, nervousness, euphoria, behavioural changes, paranoia, antisocial behaviour.
Skin: rash, sweating, purpura.
Blood disorders: thrombocytopenia, granulocytopenia.
Urogenital: difficulty in urination, impotence, delayed ejaculation, difficulty attaining orgasm in women.
Special senses: blurred vision.

CHEM NAME	TRADE NAME	FORMULATION
isocarboxazid	MARPLAN	10mg.

Maintenance dose, 10-20mg daily.
Elderly, half the adult dose.

| phenelzine | NARDIL | 15mg. |

Initially 1 three times daily reduced to maintenance.

| trancylpromine | PARNATE | 10mg. |

One twice daily. 1 three times daily if necessary.

| | PARSTELIN | 10mg with 1mg trifluoperazine. |

Maintenance usually 1 daily.
With the addition of a phenothiazine tranquilliser.

THIOXANTHENE

Category II in most cases.
Category III if large doses are taken for a long time in a weak patient where the release of a suppression may cause great difficulties for the patient.
This is used for its antipsychotic properties in higher doses (see antipsychotic agents) where it would be considered in Category IV.

CHEM NAME	TRADE NAME	FORMULATION
flupenthixol	FLUANXOL	0.5mg, 1.0mg

1-2mg daily in the morning. Maximum of 3mg daily.
Elderly: 0.5mg daily. Maximum 2mg daily.

5-HYDROXYTRYPTAMINE REUPTAKE INHIBITOR

Category II in most cases.
Category III if large doses are taken for a long time in a weak patient where the release of a suppression may cause great difficulties for the patient.
This leads to increased levels of 5-hydroxytryptamine (a central nervous system transmitter substance) in the brain.
Contraindications:
It should not be given within two weeks of stopping treatment with MAOI.
Patients with evidence of liver or kidney insufficiency should begin treatment with a low dose and be carefully monitored. The drug itself can affect hepatic function.
Effects:
General: drowsiness.
Cardiovascular: slow pulse rate (may present as palpitations).
Gastrointestinal: nausea, constipation.
Central nervous system: headache, dizziness, convulsions.
Psychological: agitation.
Skin: rashes.
Blood: neutropenia.

CHEM NAME	TRADE NAME	FORMULATION
fluvoxamine	FAVERIN	50mg.

Usual maintenance 100-200mg daily. Maximum 300mg daily.

maprotiline	LUDIOMIL	10mg, 25mg, 50mg, 75mg.

Initially 25-75mg daily. Maximum 150mg daily.
Elderly, initially 30mg at night or 10mg three times daily.
This is the most likely antidepressant to produce convulsions.

TETRACYCLICS

Category II in most cases.
Category III if large doses are taken for a long time in a weak

patient where the release of a suppression may cause great difficulties for the patient.
Contraindications:
This drug must not be used in mania or those with severe liver disease.
Precautions:
Recovery phase of myocardial infarction, epilepsy, narrow angle glaucoma and prostatic hypertrophy.
Psychotic symptoms may be increased.
Because of the effects on the blood a full blood count must be performed every four weeks during the first three months of treatment. Patients should be told to report symptoms such as sore throat, fever which may indicate affections of the blood.
Effects:
General: drowsiness.
Gastrointestinal: jaundice.
Central nervous system: convulsions.
Psychological: hypomania.
Endocrine: gynaecomastia, nipple tenderness, secretion of breast milk.
Blood: leucopenia, aplastic anaemia, agranulocytosis. This latter effect means that it must not be used as first line. Deaths have occurred.

CHEM NAME	TRADE NAME	FORMULATION
mianserin	BOLVIDON	10mg, 20mg, 30mg.
	NORVAL	10mg, 20mg, 30mg.

Usual maintenance 30-90mg daily. Maximum 200mg daily.
Elderly: initially not more than 30mg daily.

TRIAZOLOPYRIDINE

Category II in most cases.
Category III if large doses are taken for a long time in a weak patient where the release of a suppression may cause great difficulties for the patient.
Contraindications:
Not to be given to patients who take MAOI or who have stopped them within the past two weeks.
Precautions:
Caution when taken with sedatives, antidepressant drugs and alcohol, epilepsy, kidney and liver disease.

Effects:
Cardiovascular: slow heart rate, rapid heart rate, palpitations, low blood pressure on standing, oedema.
Central nervous system: weakness, tremor, dizziness, headache, blurred vision.
Psychological: drowsiness, decreased alertness, restlessness, confusional states, insomnia.
Gastrointestinal system: dry mouth, nausea, vomiting, weight loss, constipation, diarrhoea.
Skin: rash.
Priapism can occur (painful, persistent erection of the penis). Patients developing this symptom should stop the drug immediately.

CHEM NAME	TRADE NAME	FORMULATION
trazodone	MOLIPAXIN	50mg, 100mg, 150mg

150mg daily. Maximum 600mg daily.
Elderly, initially 100mg daily. Maximum 300mg daily.

OXAZINE

Category II in most cases.
Category III if large doses are taken for a long time in a weak patient where the release of a suppression may cause great difficulties for the patient.
Contraindications:
Mania, severe liver disease, history of peptic ulcer and recent myocardial infarction.
It should not be given to people who are taking MAOI or who have stopped them in the last two weeks.
Precautions:
Care with ischaemic heart disease, congestive cardiac failure, epilepsy especially if receiving phenytoin.
The depressant effect of alcohol is increased. The patient should be specifically warned.
Effects:
General: musculoskeletal pain, weight loss.
Cardiovascular: rapid heart rate, palpitations, hypertension.
Gastrointestinal: dry mouth, nausea, headache and vomiting, constipation.
Central nervous system: ataxia, dizziness, tremor and parathesiae, migraine.

Psychological: impaired alertness, anxiety and agitation, drowsiness, confusion and insomnia. Psychotic features including hypomania and aggressive behaviour may be worsened.
Urogenital: hesitant micturition.
Skin: rashes, sweating.
Special senses: blurred vision.

CHEM NAME	TRADE NAME	FORMULATION
viloxazine	VIVALAN	50mg.

300mg daily. Maximum 400mg daily.
Elderly, initially 100mg daily.

COMMENTS:

Antidepressants are very powerful agents. They are stimulants and so cause agitation, restlessness and in severe cases psychosis. They burn up the patient leading to constipation, dryness of mouth, blurred vision and so on.

They are, conventionally, given for at least three weeks because it takes that long for the effect to begin to appear. This is not strictly true as you see people whose mood changes after a few days. Certainly changes occur before the full blood level is reached.

Withdrawal of these drugs leads to the appearance of depression perhaps with weeping and sighing. The depression may be worse than the original condition and this reflects the suppression which can occur.

Typical withdrawal symptoms include anxiety, sweating, diarrhoea, hot and cold flushes, delirium and mania.

The important thing to bear in mind is that depression often overlays another, deeper emotional state. Therefore reduction must be slow to enable time to be taken dealing with the released depressive symptoms. Appropriate help such as counselling, general support or in some cases psychotherapy may be required to help with the deeper emotional states. Sudden cessation of these drugs can lead to severe difficulties for patients and should be avoided if at all possible.

In the common situation of antidepressants and tranquillisers prescribed together it is usually better to deal with the antidepressant first. This is because antidepressants are much more powerful in their effects and withdrawal will enable other, deeper states to be seen, addressed and hopefully resolved.

Appetite Suppressants

These are used in the conventional management of obesity. They are not commonly seen nowadays and nor should they be since they lead to problems of dependence in many people.

They are usually stimulant in action and people get a definite 'buzz'. People do not like to stop it because of this 'upper' effect.

It will lead to the same overstimulation as with antidepressants such as agitation, restlessness, psychosis and hallucinations.

Withdrawal leads to the appearance therefore of depression, tiredness, apathy and low spirits. These drugs relieve these symptoms and this is why it can be difficult to persuade people to come off them.

Table of Drugs in increasing order of severity

CATEGORY II
fenfluramine
CATEGORY III (because controlled drugs and potential for addiction)
diethylpropion
mazindol
phentermine

CNS STIMULANTS

Category III.
Contraindications:
They should not be prescribed at the same time as MAOI or with other appetite suppressants. Hypersensitivity to sympathomimetic amines (see Chapter 8) is also a contraindication. Other conditions are uncontrolled thyrotoxicosis, emotional instability, history of psychiatric illness, susceptibility to drug or alcohol abuse, moderate or severe hypertension and severe cardiovascular disease.
Special precautions:
Caution with concurrent administration of anti-hypertensives, anti-diabetic agents, drugs affecting the mind and emotions and sympathomimetics.

Alcohol should be avoided and patients should be specifically told this.
Effects:
Cardiovascular: palpitations, hypertension.
Psychological: restlessness, nervousness, euphoria, agitation, insomnia, depression, psychosis and hallucinations.
Gastrointestinal: nausea and vomiting, constipation. Endocrine: gynaecomastia.
Skin: rashes.

CHEM NAME	TRADE NAME	FORMULATION
diethylproprion	TENUATE DOSPAN	75mg
One mid morning.		
	APISATE	75mg with thiamine 5mg, riboflavine 4mg, pyridoxine 2mg, nicotinamide 30mg.

A mixture of diethylproprion and vitamins B1, B2, B3 and B6. One daily.
Not for the elderly.
Controlled drugs.

mazindol	TERONAC	2mg

1 daily after breakfast.
Controlled drug.

phentermine	DUROMINE	15mg, 30mg
	IONAMIN	15mg, 30mg

15 or 30mg daily.
Controlled drugs.

SEROTONINERGIC

Category II.
These drugs are the only appetite suppressants which are not controlled drugs and although similar effects are seen they are not as severe as with the remainder. Fenfluramine is related to amphetamine. Sudden withdrawal may lead to depression, dizziness, nausea, restlessness in about 20% of patients.
Contraindications:
This is not to be used in those with epilepsy, a history of depression, drug or alcohol abuse or those taking antidepressants. It should not be used at the same time as antipsychotic agents.

Precautions:
Severe depression has been reported upon sudden cessation of treatment. This is to be expected in the case of drug which stimulates.
Hypertension may be worsened.
Effects:
General: drowsiness, sedation, shivering, teeth grinding.
Cardiovascular: hypotension, hypertension.
Central nervous system: dizziness, headache, lightheadedness.
Gastrointestinal: diarrhoea, nausea, vomiting, abdominal discomfort, dry mouth.
Psychological: insomnia, unpleasant dreams, nervousness, irritability, impaired concentration, apathy, feelings of derealisation, depression, psychosis.
Urogenital: loss of libido, impotence.
Special senses: visual disturbances.
Blood disorders.
Skin: purpura, rashes, alopecia.

CHEM NAME	TRADE NAME	FORMULATION
dexfenfluramine	ADIFAX	15mg
One twice daily.		
Not for the elderly of children.		
fenfluramine	PONDERAX Pacaps	60mg
One or two daily.		

BULKING AGENTS

Category II.
These act to 'fill people up' and so reduce appetite. They are relatively harmless but can lead to problems of flatulence, abdominal distension and discomfort.

CHEM NAME	TRADE NAME	FORMULATION
methylcellulose	CELEVAC	500mg
3 tablets with warm liquid half an hour before meals or when hungry.		
	NILSTIM	400mg with cellulose
2 with a drink 15 minutes before meals.		
sterculia	PREFIL	55% (granules)
2x5ml with water half an hour before meals.		

Tranquillisers (anxiolytics)

Tranquillisers can be divided into two main groups according to their severity of action and their indications.

The 'Major' tranquillisers are used for the treatment of psychotic illnesses. They include the phenothiazines (example, LARGACTIL).

In cases of psychosis where there is use of major tranquillisers it may be better not to accept the case. There will be a great problem with suppression of symptoms, primarily mental and emotional and unless the patient can be treated in an environment with adequate support, psychotherapy and so on, it is difficult to deal with the problems which will undoubtedly arise. See antipsychotic agents later for details.

The 'Minor' tranquillisers are the commonly prescribed drugs to relieve insomnia and anxiety. They are often given in mild cases although it is being recognised by the orthodox profession that they cause dependence. They can be very difficult to stop even when taken for short periods of time. Withdrawal symptoms may be experienced after as little as 2 weeks medication.

They are all similar in terms of their general effect on the patient. They relieve the subjective feelings of anxiety, restlessness and insomnia. There is no essential difference between those given for anxiety and those given for insomnia (hypnotics).

There is a definite withdrawal syndrome with these drugs and it has been estimated that this will be the great psychiatric problem of the next twenty years. Women are prescribed them much more commonly than men as one would expect in view of the more frequent diagnosis of neurosis and hysteria in females.

The most frequently seen chemicals are the benzodiazepines, examples of which are VALIUM and ATIVAN, and they have had a very bad press in recent years. I would stress that any tranquilliser is likely to lead to dependence and rebound symptoms on withdrawal.

There is a move in some quarters to use antidepressants with marked sedating effects or even some of the major tranquillisers for anxiety in view of the problems with the benzodiazepines. This is a recipe for disaster. There is no such thing as a drug with no side-effects, there is no such thing as a drug which may not cause dependence or lead to a withdrawal syndrome when stopped. These other drugs are more likely to cause problems because they are more powerful and this practice should be opposed whenever it is seen.

Betablockers may also be used to treat anxiety since they alleviate the symptoms due to adrenaline release. They are listed in Chapter 7. When dealing with them still reduce slowly.

BENZODIAZEPINES

Category II in most cases.
Category III if large doses are taken for a long time in a weak patient where the release of a suppression may cause great difficulties for the patient.

These are the widest used of the minor tranquillisers. They are also used intravenously in epileptic attacks and to produce relaxation/amnesia before endoscopy and dental work.

Some symptoms experienced by patients when taking these drugs are considered to be 'reactions' to the benzodiazepines. These are paradoxical aggressive outbursts, antisocial acts, talkativeness, excitement, confusion and depression with suicidal tendencies. There may be amnesia for any actions as a result of these symptoms and this is of legal importance.
Contraindications:
Acute pulmonary insufficiency or respiratory depression including patients with emphysema, chronic bronchitis and those with a current attack of asthma.
Precautions:
Intravenous use can lead to hypotension or hypertension and cardiac arrest. Amnesia is a particular effect of such use.
Effects:
The elderly are particularly susceptible.
General: drowsiness, sedation. These effects which may be manifest as lack of memory and concentration may be unnoticed by patients and can occur at extremely low doses. This is of importance in those who drive or operate machinery.
Cardiovascular: hypotension.
Central nervous system: ataxia, unsteadiness, vertigo, headache, EEG changes.
Psychological: confusion, impaired memory and verbal learning.
Gastrointestinal: dry mouth, constipation, nausea, vomiting, dysphagia, anorexia, diarrhoea, jaundice.
Blood: thrombocytopenia.

Skin: rashes.
Urogenital: changes in libido, urinary retention.
Special senses: visual disturbances.

CHEM NAME	TRADE NAME	FORMULATION
alprazolam	XANAX	0.250mg, 0.5mg.

0.25mg-0.5mg three times daily. Maximum 3mg daily.
Elderly, 0.25mg two or three times daily.

| bromazepam | LEXOTAN | 1.5mg, 3mg |

3-18mg daily. Maximum 60mg daily.
Elderly, 1.5-9mg daily.

| chlor- | LIBRIUM | 5mg, 10mg, 25mg |
| diazepoxide | TROPIUM | 5mg, 10mg, 25mg |

Usually 30mg daily. Severe cases 40-100mg daily. Maximum 100mg daily.
Elderly, initially 5mg daily.

| clobazepam | FRISIUM | 10mg |

20-30mg daily. Maximum 60mg daily.
Elderly 20mg daily.
Also used in epilepsy at the same doses.

| clorazepate | TRANXENE | 7.5mg, 15mg |
| potassium | | |

Over 16 years 7.5-22.5mg daily.
Elderly 7.5mg daily.

diazepam	ALUPRAM	2mg, 5mg, 10mg
	ATENSINE	2mg, 5mg, 10mg
	SOLIS	2mg, 5mg
	TENSIUM	2mg, 5mg, 10mg
	VALIUM	2mg, 5mg, 10mg

6-30mg daily. Usual dosage is 2mg three times daily.
Elderly, 3-15mg daily.
This may cause the development of gynaecomastia in men.

| flunitrazepam | ROHYPNOL | 1mg |

Hypnotic.
½-1 at bedtime.
Elderly, ½ at bedtime.

| flurazepam | DALMANE | 15mg, 30mg |

Hypnotic.
15-30mg at bedtime.
Elderly, 15mg at bedtime.

| loprazolam | DORMONOCT | 1mg |

Hypnotic.
1-2 at bedtime.
Elderly, up to 1 at bedtime.

lorazepam	ALMAZINE	1mg, 2.5mg
	ATIVAN	1mg, 2.5mg

1-4mg daily.
Elderly, 0.5-2mg daily.

lormetazepam	generic only	0.5mg, 1.0mg

Hypnotic.
1mg at night.
Elderly, 0.5mg at night.

medazepam	NOBRIUM	5mg, 10mg

15-40mg daily.
Elderly, 5-20mg daily.

nitrazepam	MOGADON	5mg
	NITRADOS	5mg
	REMNOS	5mg, 10mg
	SOMNITE	2.5mg per 5ml suspension
	SUREM	5mg
	UNISOMNIA	5mg

Hypnotic.
5-10mg at night.
Elderly, 2.5mg to 5mg at night.

oxazepam	OXANID	10mg, 15mg, 30mg

15-30mg three or four times daily. In severe cases 60mg three times daily.
Elderly, 10-20mg three to four times daily.

temazepam	NORMISON	10mg, 20mg

Hypnotic.
10-30mg at night. Severe cases, maximum of 60mg if required.
Elderly 10mg at night.

triazolam	HALCION	0.125mg, 0.25mg

Hypnotic.
0.25mg at night.
Elderly, 0.125mg at night.
This has been implicated in causing a collection of symptoms including depersonalisation, derealisation, anxiety, depression, attacks of amnesia and aggression, paranoid feelings, altered pain threshold, nausea. The depression is described as being very severe and is only alleviated by stopping the drug. It may be related to the original dosages of around 1mg.
Note: licence revoked 1991 due to fears about its safety.

COMMENTS:

These are the commonly used tranquillisers and many millions of prescriptions are given each year. They very rapidly produce a state of dependency (within months) and withdrawal will often produce symptoms.

ATIVAN has a particularly bad name at the moment but there is little to choose between them.

WITHDRAWAL SYMPTOMS.

These are now well recognised. The severity of the manifestation depends upon the patient. However large doses used over a long time are more likely to lead to the severe withdrawal symptoms.

General: sweating, restlessness, generalised aches and pains.

Gastrointestinal: unpleasant taste, diarrhoea, nausea, dry retching.

Central nervous system: convulsions, parasthesiae.

Psychological: agitation, hallucinations, depression, nervousness, rebound insomnia, irritability, extreme sensitivity to noise and light, confusion.

It occurs even after taking 'normal' doses for a short period of time.

There have been many reports of the difficulties patients face when reducing these drugs. It is important to do this slowly. This may mean reducing the amount of drug by the merest fraction each time.

Support of family, friends and self-help groups is invaluable but the major source of help for the actual symptoms is going to be from effective treatment by alternative medicine. Acupuncture and homoeopathy have proven track-records in helping such patients. With such help it is possible to have less problems and side-effects and for the process to take less time. However these can be very difficult cases and so take care to reduce slowly and deal with each release as and when it happens. As the patient becomes stronger the process becomes smoother.

BARBITURATES

Category III.

There are other formulations not listed here which are only used for epilepsy.

They are all controlled drugs and are used in the treatment of intractable insomnia. They are very much less frequently used than 20 or 30 years ago since the advent of the benzodiazepines.

They cause addiction very readily and are more commonly seen as part of the illegal drug scene where they are taken as 'downers' often with 'speed' or amphetamines.

There is a well described withdrawal syndrome of anxiety, tremor, restlessness, weakness, gastrointestinal symptoms, delirium and convulsions.

Contraindications:

History of porphyria and those with uncontrolled pain. They should not be prescribed to children, young adults, the elderly, the debilitated or those with a history of drug or alcohol abuse.

Precautions:

Depression of respiration occurs much more than with the benzodiazepines and so use in patients with breathlessness and acute or chronic respiratory disease is potentially very dangerous. Care must be exercised in those with hepatic impairment.

Effects:

General: drowsiness, sedation, 'hangover' symptoms.

Cardiovascular: palpitations.

Gastrointestinal: changes in liver function tests.

Central nervous system: ataxia, vertigo, pain.

Psychological: excitement, confusion, memory impairment.

Skin: hypersensitive reactions especially in those with asthma or nettle rash.

CHEM NAME	TRADE NAME	FORMULATION
amylobarbitone	AMYTAL	30mg, 50mg, 100mg, 200mg
Hypnotic. 100-200mg at bedtime. Controlled drug.		
amylobarbitone sodium	SODIUM AMYTAL	60mg, 200mg
Hypnotic. 60-200mg at night. Controlled drug.		
butobarbitone	SONERYL	100mg
Hypnotic. 1-2 at bedtime. Controlled drug.		
quinalbarbitone	SECONAL	50mg, 100mg
Hypnotic. 50-100mg at bedtime.		
	TUINAL	equal parts of

quinalbarbitone with
amylobarbitone —
100mg

Hypnotic.
100-200mg at bedtime.

NON-BENZODIAZEPINE TRANQUILLISER

Category II.
Category III if large doses are taken for a long time in a weak patient where the release of a suppression may cause great difficulties for the patient.
This is a new drug which is not related chemically to the older benzodiazepines. There are some claims that it may not be addictive therefore. This is nonsense. Any drug which has such effects on the mental and emotional levels must be likely to cause dependence and the appearance of withdrawal symptoms when stopped.
Contraindications:
Epilepsy or cases of severe liver or kidney disease.
Special precautions:
History of liver or kidney impairment.
Effects:
Cardiovascular: rapid heart rate, palpitations, chest pain.
Central nervous system: dizziness, headache.
Psychological: nervousness, confusion, fatigue.
Gastrointestinal: dry mouth.

CHEM NAME	TRADE NAME	FORMULATION
buspirone	BUSPAR	5mg

1 two or three times daily. Maximum 9 daily.

SEDATIVES

There are many different types with different actions and problems. Some have been in use for many years such as chloral hydrate. Others are of very recent origin.

CHLORAL HYDRATE

Category II.
Category III if large doses are taken for a long time in a weak patient where the release of a suppression may cause great difficulties for the patient.
Contraindications:
Marked liver or kidney impairment, severe cardiac disease, severe gastritis.
Effects:
Central nervous system: headache.
Gastrointestinal: unpleasant taste, accumulation of gas, indigestion, nausea, changes in liver function tests.
Urogenital: urinary ketones.
Psychological: excitement, delirium.
Skin: allergic reactions.
Sudden withdrawal in long-term usage may precipitate delirium.

CHEM NAME	TRADE NAME	FORMULATION
chloral hydrate	NOCTEC	500mg
Hypnotic.		
1-2 at night. Maximum 4 daily.		
	WELLDORM	414mg equivalent
1-2 at night. Maximum 2G daily.		
	WELLDORM ELIXIR	143mg/5ml
15-45ml at night. Maximum 2g daily.		

CHLORMETHIAZOLE

Category II.
Category III if large doses are taken for a long time in a weak patient where the release of a suppression may cause great difficulties for the patient.
Category IV if used in psychosis, dementia and other mental rather than emotional disorders.
Contraindications:
Acute pulmonary insufficiency such as acute asthma, chest infections and so on.
Precautions:
Chronic pulmonary insufficiency such as chronic bronchitis and emphysema and chronic liver or kidney disease.

Patients with respiratory disease may develop symptoms of agitation, restlessness and confusion — the very symptoms for which this drug is prescribed.
Effects:
General: excessive sedation, 'hangover' symptoms.
Cardiovascular: cardiac arrest.
Central nervous system: headaches.
Psychological: excitement, confusion,
Gastrointestinal disturbances.
Special senses: nasal congestion and irritation, conjunctivitis.

CHEM NAME	TRADE NAME	FORMULATION
chlormethiazole	HEMINEVRIN	250mg per 5ml syrup or as capsule (one capsule = 5ml syrup)

Hypnotic and sedative.
10ml or 2 capsules at night.
Sedation: 5ml or 1 capsule three times daily.
This drug is used particularly for severe insomnia in the elderly, for agitated confusional states, senile psychosis or to control the withdrawal symptoms seen in alcoholism.

CHLORMEZANONE

Category II.
Category III if large doses are taken for a long time in a weak patient where the release of a suppression may cause great difficulties for the patient.
Contraindications:
This drug should not be given to those already taking MAOI.
Precautions:
Kidney and liver disease.
Effects:
General: drowsiness, sedation, lethargy.
Central nervous system: dizziness, headaches, lightheadedness.
Psychological: depression.
Gastrointestinal: nausea, dryness of the mouth.
Skin: flushing, reddening, nettle rash.

CHEM NAME	TRADE NAME	FORMULATION
chlormezanone	TRANCOPAL	200mg

Hypnotic.
2 at night.
Elderly, 1 at night.

ANTIHISTAMINE

Category II.
These may be used for sedation since their common effect is to produce tiredness and drowsiness. See Chapter 8 for a fuller description.

CHEM NAME	TRADE NAME	FORMULATION
hydroxyzine	ATARAX	10mg, 25mg, 10mg/5ml

50-100mg four times daily.

promethazine	SOMINEX	20mg

Hypnotic.
1 at bedtime or up to 1 hour after going to bed.

CYCLOPYRROLONE

Category II.
Category III if large doses are taken for a long time in a weak patient where the release of a suppression may cause great difficulties for the patient.
A new tranquilliser with little information currently available.
Regard as the benzodiazepines.
Special precautions:
Close monitoring required in cases of hepatic insufficiency.
Effects:
General: drowsiness, impaired dexterity.
Gastrointestinal: metallic taste, gastrointestinal disturbances.
Psychological disturbances.
Allergic reactions.

CHEM NAME	TRADE NAME	FORMULATION
zopiclone	ZIMOVANE	7.5mg

1 at night. 2 if necessary.
Elderly, initially half a tablet.

CARBAMATE TRANQUILLISER

Category II.
Category III if large doses are taken for a long time in a weak patient where the release of a suppression may cause great difficulties for the patient.
Contraindications:
Acute intermittent porphyria and alcoholism.
Precautions:
Impaired liver or kidney function, history of epilepsy or depression.
Effects:
General: drowsiness.
Cardiovascular: hypotension.
Central nervous system: parasthesiae.
Psychological: excitement, poor concentration.
Blood disorders: thrombocytopenia, pancytopenia, aplastic anaemia.
Allergy: hypersensitivity reactions.

CHEM NAME	TRADE NAME	FORMULATION
meprobamate	EQUANIL	200mg, 400mg

400mg three times daily and at bedtime.
Elderly, 200mg three times daily.
Controlled drug.

PHENOTHIAZINE-LIKE

Category II unless given for psychotic disorders when Category IV is more appropriate.
Contraindications:
They should not be given to people who are taking MAOI or who have taken them within the past three weeks.
Effects:
General: drowsiness.
Central nervous system: dizziness.
Gastrointestinal: dry mouth.

CHEM NAME	TRADE NAME	FORMULATION
oxypertine	INTEGRIN	10mg

1 three or four times daily. Maximum 6 daily.

Case Examples

CASE 1

A woman of 55 years suffered a bereavement some 30 years ago and since then had experienced depression periodically with sadness, weeping and feelings of unhappiness. Whenever this happened she was given antidepressants and had been taking them continuously for the past 15 years.

Other symptoms were anxiety, feelings of panic, insomnia, sweating, palpitations, poor memory and concentration.

Medication:

> MOGADON 5mg at night.
> VALIUM 5mg three times daily.
> ANAFRANIL 25mg two at night.
> INDERAL 10mg three times daily.

Listed in order of increasing strength.

This picture is commonly seen with psychoactive drugs. The original symptoms of depression have been suppressed by antidepressants (ANAFRANIL) which cause anxiety and panics. With long-term usage these anxiety symptoms become more pronounced and may need the addition of tranquillisers (VALIUM), hypnotics (MOGADON) and even betablockers (INDERAL). In the end the patient will have no idea what is going on emotionally since any feeling is blocked by a drug and their effects further complicate the picture.

It is a difficult situation to deal with but begin with the most powerful agent first. The order of reduction should be strongest to weakest so that support is given by the weaker drugs.

As each drug is reduced and then stopped you would expect to see a flareup of the symptoms suppressed by that drug. Therefore, the sedating drugs — INDERAL, VALIUM, MOGADON — , as they are reduced, lead to the appearance of anxiety, restlessness and insomnia. The INDERAL prevents any feelings of ill-ease as it blocks almost completely the adrenaline response. Therefore, this must be removed if the patient is to regain contact with her emotional state.

The antidepressant as it is removed will lead to the appearance of depression manifest often as sadness, weeping and feelings of loss. Again, these feelings need to be resolved before moving on either to further reductions or to total cessation.

In this particular case it took over 3 years to remove the drugs completely. There were other difficulties since the patient lived on her own and had little support from friends or family. Acupuncture treatment was supplemented with counselling and relaxation sessions.

The length of time taken to attain a drug-free existence reflects the depth of the neurosis and the duration of drug treatment (in this case over 30 years).

CASE 2

A man of 43 years had, for the past 4 years, been taking tranquillisers since having panic attacks as a result of stressful situations at home and work. He went to his GP then who put him on VALIUM and had not been able to stop since.

Medication:

> VALIUM 17.5mg daily on weekdays and 12.5mg at weekends.

His main symptoms were those of panic, feeling of a lump in the throat, feelings of not being able to breathe properly. These were always present although tolerable. Whenever he reduced the VALIUM they became more noticeable and accompanied by a fear of indeterminate origin eventually blind panic.

This is one of the problems of this group of drugs. The Chinese view is that fear is rooted in the kidneys and these drugs deplete the kidneys energetically causing fear and panic. Therefore patients are in a Catch-22 situation — they cannot stop the drug because the feelings of panic are intolerable and yet continuation leads to further damage and the development of ever more severe anxiety and panic.

The approach is to attempt to resolve some of the emotional state so that the drug can be reduced. Reduction will reveal more emotion to be resolved. This is a step-wise process which will have its own pace in each individual.

CASE 3

This case shows the problems which can ensue through the use of drugs which are much too powerful for the situation.

A young man of 23 years had suffered from anxiety since childhood although it had always been manageable and he had developed his own ways of coping with it.

At the age of 18 when taking examinations at school his

anxiety became more of a problem and he was prescribed STELAZINE first followed by SERENACE. The latter drug caused rigidity of muscles with a locked jaw — typical of the Parkinsonian-like effects it is noted for. This event frightened him severely and his anxiety was considerably worse. He was subsequently given ATIVAN 2.5mg three times daily regularly which only helped to a minor degree.

This use of powerful antipsychotic agents for anxiety is indefensible but is increasingly seen since doctors are waking up to the problems associated with the benzodiazepines.

Treatment was prolonged over a year but at the end of that time he reached the stage where his ATIVAN had been withdrawn. He was still having problems with anxiety but it was manageable and he was able to return to his college studies.

ATIVAN at this level is a high dosage and it shows the degree of problem he had at this time. Reduction is preferable by stages of 1mg tablets which are available rather in steps of 2.5mg.

Neuroleptics and Antipsychotic Agents

These all fall into Category IV as stated in Chapter 3. There are various groups and they are all used in the treatment of severe psychological disorders such as schizophrenia where thought disorders, hallucinations and delusions are present. They can also be used in demented or confused patients where these symptoms are a feature.

I have included drugs used in the treatment of manic depression such as lithium although strictly speaking they are not considered to be antipsychotic drugs.

Adverse effects are commonly seen and interestingly, their occurrence is not necessarily dose related. The main problems patients experience are behavioural worsening and neurological symptoms.

I have included all the antipsychotics together as a group because they have very similar effects.

Contraindications:

Comatose states, marked cerebral atherosclerosis, phaeochromocytoma, renal failure, liver failure, severe cardiac impairment, severe depression, bone marrow disease, concurrent use or withdrawal of large doses of sedatives (including alcohol, barbiturates, opiates). High dose therapy is not to be used in children or the elderly.

Precautions:
Liver disease, renal failure, Parkinson's disease, phaeochromocytoma, thyrotoxicosis, epilepsy and conditions predisposing
to epilepsy, e.g. brain damage, alcohol withdrawal.
Because blood can be affected it is important to perform blood
counts on the appearance of symptoms of infection such as
fever, sore throat or enlarged lymph glands.
Effects:
In delusional states the therapeutic response may not be immediate and conversely when the drug is stopped it may take
several weeks or months for the symptoms to appear.
Effects in children are unpredictable and sudden infant death
may occur.
General: sedation especially in the elderly, weight gain is seen
in virtually all patients.
Cardiovascular: rapid heart rate, postural hypotension especially in the elderly, oedema, ECG changes. Cardiac arrhythmias are more likely in the elderly, if concurrently using
tricyclic antidepressants, in those with pre-existing heart disease. A pre-treatment ECG is a sensible precaution. Some
cardiac arrhythmias may be fatal.
Respiratory: Pulmonary embolism, suppression of the gag and
cough reflexs. Regular examination of the gag reflex is recommended in those with tardive dyskinesia (see central nervous
system effects).
Gastrointestinal: dry mouth, nausea, loss of appetite, dyspepsia, constipation, liver function test changes, jaundice.
Central nervous system: headache, dizziness, EEG changes,
epileptic fits.
Extrapyramidal effects which include:
i) acute dystonic reaction.
Within 1–2 days of starting treatment or after a dose increase
there is sudden onset of muscular spasms such as opisthotonos
and torticollis. This is more likely in men than women and in
the younger patient.
ii) akathisia.
Restlessness of the legs with anxiety and mood alteration. The
restlessness may bve of a variable degree from inability to sit or
stand still to severe behavioural disorders.
iii) Parkinsonism.
This is indistinguishable from Parkinsonism due to any other
cause.
iv) Tardive dyskinesia.
These are spontaneous irregular movements performed in a

repetitive manner. They include chewing, licking, smacking of the lips, tongue protrusion, tongue movements, rocking movements, akathisia. It typically occurs after long term treatment but can develop in under a year. It is seen in up to 65% of patients.

TD, as it is known, is commoner in women and the elderly. The incidence may also be increased in those with emotional disturbances and a history of alcohol abuse or treatment with electroconvulsive therapy.

Antiparkinsonian drugs increase the symptoms.

Whether TD is alleviated by drug withdrawal is a matter of debate. In my experience many patients continue to have residual problems which are very resistant to any form of treatment. This may reflect a degree of CNS structual damage.

Psychological: mental dullness, feeling of being slowed down, depression, excitement, agitation, insomnia, worsening of the psychosis, confusional states, catatonic states.

Endocrine: gynaecomastia, secretion of breast milk in non-pregnant women, scanty or no periods, false positive pregnancy test.

Urogenital: urinary retention, incontinence, dysuria, impaired sexual function such as impairment of ejaculation and erection, priapism.

Blood: agranulocytosis, thrombocytopenia, haemolytic anaemia, leucopenia, neutropenia.

Skin: urticaria, photosensitivity, skin discolouration, rashes, hirsutism.

Special senses: blurred vision, deposits in the cornea or lens, optic atrophy, blue-green colour blindness, night blindness, transient myopia.

BUTYROPHENONE

Category IV.

CHEM NAME	TRADE NAME	FORMULATION
benperidol 0.25–1.5mg daily.	ANQUIL	0.25mg
droperidol 5–20mg three to six times daily.	DROLEPTAN	10mg, 1mg/ml
haloperidol	DOZIC FORTUNAN	1mg/ml, 2mg/ml 0.5mg, 1.5mg, 5mg, 10mg, 20mg

| | HALDOL | 5mg, 10mg, 2mg/ml, 10mg/ml |
| | SERENACE | 0.5mg, 1.5mg, 10mg, 20mg, 2mg/ml |

Psychoses, initially 0.5–5mg two or three times daily. Maximum 200mg daily. Maintenance dose usually 5–10mg daily.
Elderly, initially 0.5–2mg daily.
Anxiety, 0.5mg twice daily.

| trifluperidol | TRIPERIDOL | 0.5mg, 1mg |

0.5mg daily. Maximum 6–8mg daily.

THIOXANTHENE

Category IV.
These are related to the phenothiazines.

CHEM NAME	TRADE NAME	FORMULATION
flupenthixol	DEPIXOL	3mg

1–3 twice daily. Maximum 6 daily.

| zuclopenthixol | CLOPIXOL | 2mg, 10mg, 25mg |

Maintenance, 20–50mg daily. Maximum 150mg daily.

DIPHENYLBUTYLPIPERIDINE

Category IV.

CHEM NAME	TRADE NAME	FORMULATION
fluspirilene	REDEPTIN	Given as injection weekly.
pimozide	ORAP	2mg, 4mg, 10mg

2–20mg daily.

PHENOTHIAZINES

Category IV.

CHEM NAME	TRADE NAME	FORMULATION
chlorpromazine	LARGACTIL	10mg, 25mg, 50mg, 100mg, 25/5ml

Maintenance, usually 75–100mg daily.

fluphenazine	MODECATE	Given as injection every 2–5 weeks.
	MODITEN	1mg, 2.5mg, 5mg

In anxiety and tension, 1–2mg daily.
Psychotic states, 2.5–10mg daily. Maximum 20mg daily.

metho-trimeprazine	NOZINAN	25mg

25–50mg daily if ambulant. 100–200mg daily if not.

oxypertine	INTEGRIN	40mg

1 two or three times daily. Maximum 300mg daily.

pericyazine	NEULACTIL	2.5mg, 10mg, 25mg, 10mg/5ml

Initially 15–75mg daily.
Elderly, initially 15–30mg daily.

perphenazine	FENTAZIN	2mg, 4mg

12mg daily. Maximum 24mg daily.

pipothiazine	PIPORTIL DEPOT	Given by injection every 4 weeks

pro-chlorperazine	STEMETIL	5mg, 25mg, 5mg/5ml

Minor mental disturbances, 15–20mg daily. Maximum of 40mg daily.
Schizophrenia, 75–100mg daily.
This drug is also used in the treatment of nausea, vomiting.

promazine	SPARINE	50mg/5ml

100–200mg four times daily.
Elderly, half the adult dose or 25–50mg for restlessness.

thioridazine	MELLERIL	10mg, 25mg, 50mg, 100mg, 25mg/5ml, 100mg/5ml

30–100mg daily, increasing to 600mg daily.
This drug may lead to retinal disease which may seriously affect vision.

trifluoperazine	STELAZINE	1mg, 5mg.

5mg twice daily. The dose is increased further by 5mg increments then reduced to maintenance dose.

	STELAZINE SPANSULES	2mg, 10mg, 15mg sustained-release

15mg daily.

SUBSTITUTED BENZAMIDE

Category IV.

CHEM NAME	TRADE NAME	FORMULATION
sulpiride	DOLMATIL	200mg
	SULPITIL	200mg

Over 14 years, initially 400–800mg daily. Maximum 1800mg daily.

DIBENZOXAZEPINE

Category IV.

A very new antipsychotic agent used when patients are unresponsive to other antipsychotics. It may be that the effects are in fact very similar to the others but information is sparse at this time.

Contraindications:

Not to be used in comatose states or drug-induced depression.

Precautions:

Epilepsy, cardiovascular disease, glaucoma, urinary retention. Patients should be warned to report signs of infection such as fever, sore throat or lymphatic gland enlargement because of the possible effects on the blood.

Effects:

General: weakness, drowsiness, impaired dexterity.

Respiratory: breathlessness.

Cardiovascular: rapid heart rate, palpitations, low or high blood pressure.

Central nervous system: dizziness, muscle twitching, Parkinsonian-like symptoms, headache. The full extent of CNS effects are not yet known.

Gastrointestinal system: nausea, vomiting.

Psychological: confusion.

Blood: agranulocytosis (clozapine).

Skin: rash.

CHEM NAME	TRADE NAME	FORMULATION
clozapine	CLOZARIL	25mg, 100mg
loxapine	LOXAPAC	10mg, 25mg, 50mg.

Initially 20–50 daily. Maximum 250mg daily.

IMINOSTILBENE

Category IV.
This is quoted as being used for patients with manic depression who are unresponsive to lithium therapy. I have never seen it used in this way and it is an unusual approach. It is much more commonly seen used in epilepsy and the drug is covered in more detail in Chapter 10.

CHEM NAME	TRADE NAME	FORMULATION
carbamazepine	TEGRETOL	100mg, 200mg, 400mg
400mg–600mg daily. Maximum 1.6G daily.		

LITHIUM COMPOUNDS

These are all Category IV drugs.
Typically, reduction of dosage leads to reappearance of the symptoms of mania or depression four weeks after the drug has been stopped completely. This can mean that all appears to be well until there is a sudden flare-up of the clinical picture.
Contraindications:
Renal disease, cardiovascular disease and Addison's disease.
Precautions:
Periodic routine clinical monitoring is essential in all patients and there should be regular assessment of renal function, urine analysis, thyroid and cardiac function.
All patients should be given details of the symptoms of lithium toxicity. They should also be told to report excessive urination or thirst, nausea and vomiting and any other conditions which lead to dehydration.
Elderly people are particularly liable to develop lithium toxicity.
Warnings:
Long term treatment may lead to renal damage and impairment of renal function.
Effects:
Central nervous system: vertigo, muscle weakness, fine hand tremors. Psychological: dazed feelings, impaired thought processes. Gastrointestinal: nausea, mild thirst.
Urogenital: polyuria.
Long term treatment is often associated with disturbed thyroid function particularly goitre, hypothyroidism or thyrotoxicosis.

CHEM NAME	TRADE NAME	FORMULATION
lithium	CAMCOLIT	250mg, 400mg
carbonate	LISKONUM	450mg
	PHASAL	300mg
	PRIADEL	200mg, 400mg
lithium citrate	LITAREX	564mg

The dose of lithium given to patients will vary with each individual case because the optimum is decided by levels of lithium in the blood. Therefore, treatment is monitored by regular checks on the blood every month when the patient is stabilised.

COMMENTS:

The antipsychotic agents are used in the treatment of severe psychological disorders such as schizophrenia, delusional states and so on. They cause many problems for the patient because of their powerful action and they reflect the seriousness with which current society views such symptoms.

Tardive dyskinesia is more common in those who have had long-term treatment but can occur after low doses for short periods. It can be irreversible. It can be worsened or precipitated by giving anti-Parkinsonism drugs.

Short term dyskinesias can be seen after abrupt withdrawal of the drugs.

The conventional medical aim is to control the symptoms of the psychosis so there are no hard and fast rules about the ideal dosage. There is clearly room here for practitioners of alternative medicine to offer help in an appropriate set-up so that such agents can be withdrawn if improvement occurs. Such treatment would clearly risk the reappearance of the symptoms of delusion, hallucination, thought disorders and the like, so typical of schizophrenia and related disorders.

This reappearance of symptoms means that out-patient treatment is very difficult. Patients require a lot of help and support not just by one therapy such as homoeopathy or acupuncture but also perhaps by psychotherapy, counselling and so on. I do believe that it is possible to offer this sort of approach. However I would not routinely treat patients in the context of out-patient practice.

7   CARDIOVASCULAR SYSTEM

Hypertension

Conventional treatment is by means of diuretics and hypotensive agents — drugs which lower blood pressure. Various hypotensive drugs are currently available but betablockers are by far the commonest prescribed.

Other drugs are used according to the doctor's personal preference or where the betablockers are contraindicated. These others tend to be older drugs which have been in use for many years.

CENTRAL ALPHA AGONISTS

Category II drug.
There are several examples of this drug available.

METHYL DOPA

The important effects relate to postural hypotension — that is low blood pressure when standing. It is common especially in the elderly and leads to dizziness, lightheadedness and falling perhaps with loss of consciousness.

Contraindications:
Active liver disease such as acute hepatitis, active cirrhosis and depression.

Precautions:
Any patient who develops fever, abnormality in liver function or jaundice should stop treatment. The drug may be resumed if the symptoms and signs are unrelated to the drug. I would imagine it is very difficult to be absolutely certain about this. Fatal liver damage has occurred.

Effects:
General: sedation, drowsiness, weakness, muscle pains, joint pains.
Cardiovascular: slow pulse rate, worsening of angina pectoris, postural hypotension, oedema, rise in blood pressure.
Gastrointestinal: nausea, vomiting, distension, constipation, flatus, diarrhoea, colitis, dryness of mouth, sore or 'black' tongue, pancreatitis, enlargement of the salivary glands.
Hepatic: jaundice, abnormal liver function tests, hepatitis.
Central nervous system: headache, paraesthesiae, worsening of

Parkinson's disease, Bell's palsy, involuntary movements, dizziness, lightheadedness.

Psychological: nightmares, impaired mental alertness, mild
psychoses, forgetfulness, nightmares, depression.

Endocrine: breast enlargement, gynaecomastia, amenorrhoea,
secretion of milk from the breast, decreased libido.

Blood: haemolytic anaemia which may be fatal, granulocytopenia, thrombocytopenia.

Allergic: drug-related fever, inflammation of heart muscle and
pericardium.

Urogenital: decreased libido, impotence, failure of ejaculation,
dark urine.

Skin: eczema-like rashes.

Special senses: nasal stuffiness.

CHEM NAME	TRADE NAME	FORMULATION
methyldopa	ALDOMET	125mg, 250mg, 500mg, 250mg/5ml
	DOPAMET	125mg, 250mg, 500mg
	MEDOMET	250mg, 500mg

250mg two or three times daily. maximum 3G daily.
Elderly: 125mg three times daily is often sufficient.

	HYDROMET	250mg with 15mg hydrochlorothiazide

1 twice daily. Maximum 12 daily.
With the addition of a thiazide diuretic.

BETABLOCKER

These drugs are always considered to be in Category III
irrespective of their indicated use.

These are probably the most widely used agents for the treatment of hypertension. They are also used for migraine, anxiety
attacks, hyperthyroidism and to control or prevent the pain of
angina pectoris.

They block the receptors which respond to adrenaline and
adrenaline-like substances and result in the relief of subjective
feelings of anxiety and panic. They will reduce the work done
by the heart and lead to slowing of the pulse and reduction in
blood pressure. They also have an effect in painful conditions
such as migraine. The mechanism here is not well understood
conventionally.

Because these receptors are in many different types of tissue, effects are wide-ranging. The effect on the lungs is to produce wheezing in susceptible individuals. Deaths have occurred in some affected in this way. Although there are betablockers which are claimed to be 'cardio-selective' people can still wheeze with these and there are dangers in giving any betablocker to a patient with asthma or other wheezing disease eg chronic bronchitis.

They are being increasingly used by people who need to have a calm approach to situations of stress so they are used by public speakers or by athletes who require steady hands. For this reason they are on the banned list of substances for pistol shooting and snooker.

Contraindications:

Certain arrhythmias, history of wheezing, after prolonged fasting and in patients with diabetes mellitus (because these drugs block the adrenaline response patients cannot detect when they become hypoglycaemic — a potentially fatal situation in a diabetic).

Precautions:

Cardiac failure can be precipitated or made worse by these drugs. The dose should be reduced if the heart rate is slow.

They should not be stopped suddenly if there is ischaemic heart disease. What this means in practice is that where these agents have been given for a prolonged period of time (over several months) they should be reduced slowly because sudden withdrawal can lead to a coronary thrombosis. Since many people have ischaemic heart disease to some degree it seems sensible to reduce slowly even in people who have received this drug for migraine or anxiety.

Effects:

General: tiredness, lack of energy.

Cardiovascular: cold extremities, slow pulse rate, hypotension, chest pain, exacerabation of Raynaud's phenomenon.

Gastrointestinal: nausea, diarrhoea, dyspepsia, constipation.

Central nervous system: parasthesiae in the hands.

Psychological: insomnia.

Urogenital: impotence.

Skin: rashes.

Special senses: dry eyes, conjunctivitis, visual disturbances.

CHEM NAME	TRADE NAME	FORMULATION
acebutolol	SECTRAL	100mg, 200mg, 400mg

Hypertension: up to 400mg twice daily.
Angina: 200mg twice daily. Maximum 1.2G daily.

| | SECADREX | 200mg with 12.5mg hydrochlorothiazide |

Hypertension: 1–2 daily.
With the addition of a thiazide diuretic.

atenolol	ANTIPRESSAN50mg,	100mg
	TENORMIN LS	50mg
	TENORMIN	100mg, 25mg/ml
	TOTAMOL	
	VASATEN	

50–100mg daily.
Hypertension: 50–100mg daily.
Angina: 100mg daily.

| | KALTEN | 50mg with 25mg hydrochlorothiazide 2.5mg amiloride |

1 daily.
With the addition of a thiazide diuretic and a low potency diuretic.

| | TENORET 50 | 50mg with 12.5mg chlorthalidone |

1 daily.
With the addition of a thiazide diuretic.

| | TENORETIC | 100mg with 25mg chlorthalidone |

1 daily.
With the addition of a thiazide diuretic.

| | BETA-ADALAT | 50mg with 20mg nifedipine |
| | TENIF | 50mg with 20mg nifedipine |

Hypertension and angina: 1–2 daily.
Elderly, maximum of 1 daily.
With the addition of calcium antagonist.

| betaxolol | KERLONE | 20mg |

Hypertension: 1 daily.

bisoprolol	EMCOR	10mg
	EMCOR LS	5mg
	MONOCOR	5mg, 10mg

Hypertension and angina: usually 10mg daily; maximum 20mg daily.

| carteolol | CARTROL | 10mg |

Angina: 10–30mg daily.

| metoprolol | BETALOC | 50mg, 100mg |
| | LOPRESOR | 50mg, 100mg |

Hypertension: 100mg daily. Maximum 400mg daily.
Angina: usually 50–100mg two or three times daily.

| | BETALOC SA | 200mg sustained-release |
| | LOPRESOR SR | 200mg sustained-release |

Hypertension and angina: sustained-release form. 1–2 daily.

| | CO-BETALOC | 100mg with 12.5mg |
| | | hydrochlorothiazide |

1–3 daily.
With the addition of a thiazide diuretic.

| | CO-BETALOC SA | 200mg with 25mg |
| | | hydrochlorothiazide |

Sustained release form of metoprolol. Usually 1 daily.
With the addition of a thiazide diuretic.

| | LOPRESORETIC | 100mg with 12.5mg |
| | | chlorthalidone |

1 daily. If necessary 3–4 daily.
With the addition of a thiazide diuretic.

| | METOROS | 190mg |

A different salt of metoprolol and so is NOT interchangeable with the above forms of metoprolol. 1 or 2 daily.

| | METOROS LS | 95mg |

As the above but a sustained-release form. Initially 1 daily.

| nadolol | CORGARD | 40mg, 80mg |

Hypertension: 80–240mg daily.
Angina: 40–240mg daily.

| | CORGARETIC 40 | 40mg with 5mg |
| | | bendrofluazide |

1–2 daily.
With the addition of a thiazide diuretic.

| | CORGARETIC 80 | 80mg with 5mg |
| | | bendrofluazide |

1–2 daily.
With the addition of a thiazide diuretic.

oxprenolol	APSOLOX	20mg, 40mg, 80mg, 160mg
	OXYPRENIX	
	TRASICOR	20mg, 40mg, 80mg, 160mg

Hypertension: 80mg twice daily. Maximum of 480mg daily.
Angina: 40–160mg three times daily. Maximum of 480mg daily.

| | SLOW-PREN | 160mg sustained-release |
| | SLOW-TRASICOR | 160mg sustained-release |

Hypertension and angina: 1–3 daily.

| | TRASIDREX | 160mg with 0.25mg |

cyclopenthiazide

1 daily. 2 or more daily may be required.
With the addition of a thiazide diuretic.

penbutolol   LASIPRESSIN   40mg with 20mg
                                     frusemide

1–2 daily.
With the addition of a high potency diuretic.

pindolol   VISKEN   5mg, 15mg
Hypertension: 10–15mg daily. Maximum 45mg daily.
Angina: 2.5–5mg up to three times daily.

                  VISKALDIX   10mg with 5mg
                                     clopamide

1 daily. Maximum of 3 daily.
With the addition of a diuretic.
This is particularly likely to cause a resting tremor.

propranolol   ANGILOL   10mg, 40mg, 80mg, 160mg
                  APSOLOL   10mg, 40mg, 80mg, 160mg
                  BERKOLOL   10mg, 40mg, 80mg, 160mg
                  CARDINOL
                  INDERAL   40mg, 80mg, 160mg
Hypertension: 160–320mg daily.
Angina: 40mg two or three times daily. Maximum 480mg daily.

                  BEDRANOL SR   160mg sustained-release
                  HALF INDERAL LA   80mg sustained-release
                  INDERAL LA   160mg sustained-release
Hypertension: 160mg daily increasing by 80mg until control achieved.
Angina: Up to 160mg daily.

                  INDERETIC   80mg with 2.5mg
                                     bendrofluazide

1 twice daily.
With the addition of a thiazide diuretic.

                  INDEREX   160mg with 5mg
                                     bendrofluazide

1 daily.
With the addition of a thiazide diuretic.

sotalol   BETA-CARDONE   40mg, 80mg, 200mg
Hypertension and angina: usually 200–600mg daily.

                  SOTACOR   80mg, 160mg
Hypertension: 160–320mg daily.
Angina: 160mg daily.

                  SOTAZIDE   160mg with 25mg
                                     hydrochlorothiazide

1–2 daily.
With the addition of a thiazide diuretic.

                  TOLERZIDE   80mg with 12.5mg

hydrochlorothiazide
1 daily.
With the addition of a thiazide diuretic.

| timolol | BETIM | 10mg |
| | BLOCADREN | 10mg |

Hypertension and angina: maintenance 10–30mg daily. Maximum 60mg daily.

	MODUCREN	10mg with 25mg
		hydrochlorothiazide
		2.5mg amiloride

1–2 daily.
With the addition of a thiazide diuretic and a low potency diuretic.

| | PRESTIM | 10mg with 2.5mg |
| | | bendrofluazide |

1–4 daily.
With the addition of a thiazide diuretic.

ALPHA AND BETABLOCKER

Category III drugs.
There is some relationship with betablockers but these drugs also block alpha receptors.
Contraindications:
Certain cardiac arrhythmias, severely slow pulse or where hypotension has been present for some time.
Precautions:
Poor cardiac function, asthma or history of wheezing, those with ischaemic heart disease should not stop treatment suddenly.
Effects:
General: tiredness, lethargy.
Cardiovascular: postural hypotension, ankle oedema.
Gastrointestinal: nausea, vomiting, epigastric pain.
Central nervous system: dizziness, headache, tremor, perioral numbness, parasthesiae of scalp.
Psychological: depression.
Urogenital: acute retention of urine, difficulty of urination.
Allergy: fever, rash, itching, oedema, breathlessness.
Skin: sweating.
Special senses: nasal congestion.

CHEM NAME	TRADE NAME	FORMULATION
labetalol	LABROCOL	100mg, 200mg, 400mg
	TRANDATE	50mg, 100mg, 200mg, 400mg

Hypertension and angina: 100–200mg twice daily. Maximum 2.4G daily.
Elderly: 50mg twice daily.

ADRENERGIC NEURONE BLOCKERS

Category III drugs.
These are an older type of drug and are not often used nowadays.
Contraindications:
Patients should not also take sympathomimetic agents such as adrenaline, amphetamine, appetite suppressants.
Precautions:
Cases of cerebral or coronary vascular disease, renal impairment.
Effects:
General: The effects of this group of agents are more marked when standing. So faintness, sweating, muscle tiredness and headache may occur with sudden changes of posture, excessive exercise and extremes of temperature.
Cardiovascular: Hypotension especially postural and after exercise.
Slow heart rate (may manifest as palpitations).
Gastrointestinal: dry mouth, disturbed taste, diarrhoea
Central nervous system: tremor, parasthesiae.
Urogenital: disturbed urination, failure of ejaculation in 25–65%, impotence.
Special senses: nasal stuffiness, photophobia.

CHEM NAME	TRADE NAME	FORMULATION
bethanidine	BENDOGEN	10mg, 50mg
	ESBATAL	10mg, 50mg

Initially 10mg three times daily; maximum 200mg daily.

debrisoquine	DECLINAX	10mg, 20mg

Initially 10–20mg once or twice daily. Maximum 120mg daily.

guanethidine	ISMELIN	10mg, 25mg

20mg daily. Increased by 10mg increments if necessary.

ACE INHIBITOR

Category III drugs.

Also used in the treatment of cardiac failure.

These should not be routinely given to those with impaired renal function, collagen vascular disease, immunosuppressant therapy. Blood disorders occur primarily in these groups.

If therapy is given in these patients then blood cell counts should be performed before treatment begins, every two weeks during the first three months of treatment and periodically thereafter.

Precautions:

Everyone considered for treatment with these drugs should have an assessment of renal function, this is minimally a urinalysis and serum urea and creatinine.

Blood changes such as neutropenia, anaemia and thrombocytopenia can occur. It should not be given routinely to people who have autoimmune disease affecting the blood vessels, those who take immunosuppressants or those with impaired renal function because neutropenia occurs mainly in these groups.

All patients should be specifically told to report any sign of infection such as sore throat, fever so that a white blood cell count can be undertaken.

Proteinuria may occur but usually this is in patients with severe hypertension or previous renal disease. Nephrotic syndrome has occurred in such patients. If the drug is given to patients with pre-existing renal disease then monthly urinary protein estimations by 'dip stick' should be performed for the first nine months of treatment.

At the start of therapy hypotension may occur. This is exaggerated in patients who have cardiac failure receiving large doses of diuretics.

Effects:

General: lymphatic gland enlargement.

Cardiovascular: hypotension, rapid heart rate which may precipitate angina in some patients, palpitations.

Respiratory: cough, wheezing.

Gastrointestinal: taste impairment which is usually reversible, weight loss, stomatitis resembling apthous ulcers, nausea, indigestion, abdominal pain, liver function abnormalities, liver damage, jaundice.

Central nervous system: parathesiae of the hands.

Blood disorders: neutropenia, thrombocytopenia, anaemia, agranulocytosis, pancytopenia.

Skin: rashes usually itchy. These are usually transient, mild and maculopapular. Some may be urticarial. Some patients have experienced itching, flushing, vesicular rash and photosensivity.

Urogenital: proteinuria, metabolic changes.

CHEM NAME	TRADE NAME	FORMULATION
captopril	ACEPRIL	12.5mg, 25mg, 50mg
	CAPOTEN	12.5mg, 25mg, 50mg

Hypertension: maintenance 25mg twice daily. Usual maximum of 50mg twice daily. In severe cases 50mg three times daily.
Cardiac failure: 25mg three times daily. Maximum 150mg daily.

	ACEZIDE	50mg with 25mg hydrochlorothiazide
	CAPOZIDE	50mg with 25mg hydrochlorothiazide

1–2 daily.
With the addition of a thiazide diuretic.

enalapril	INNOVACE	2.5mg, 5mg, 10mg, 20mg

Hypertension: usual maintenance, 10–20mg daily. Maximum 40mg daily.
Cardiac failure: usual maintenance 10–20mg daily.

lisinopril	CARACE	2.5mg, 5mg, 10mg, 20mg
	ZESTRIL	2.5mg, 5mg, 10mg, 20mg

Hypertension: maintenance of 10–20mg daily. Maximum 40mg daily.
Cardiac failure: maintenance of 5–20mg daily.

perindopril	COVERSYL	2mg, 4mg

Hypertension: 4–8mg once daily.

quinapril	ACCUPRO	5mg, 10mg, 20mg

Hypertension: 20–40mg daily. Maximum 80mg daily.
Cardiac failure: 10–20mg daily. Maximum 40mg daily. Elderly, 2.5mg daily.

ramipril	TRITACE	1.75mg, 2.5mg, 5mg

Maintenance 2.5–5mg daily. Maximum 10mg daily.

CLONIDINE

Category III drug. This is also a central alpha agonist — see page 98 for others.
Also used in lower doses as a prophylactic in migraine.

Precautions:
Withdrawal may lead to sudden rebound rise in the blood pressure and so drug reduction should be gradual. Agitation may appear upon withdrawal as well as sweating, trembling and rapid heart rate.

Those with a history of depression should be monitored closely as clonidine may produce such states.

Care also in those with Raynaud's disease, peripheral arterial disease, cerebrovascular, coronary and renal impairment.

Effects:
General: sedation, fatigue.

Cardiovascular system: fluid retention, hypotension, slow pulse rate.

Gastrointestinal: nausea, vomiting, dry mouth, anorexia, constipation, hepatitis.

Central nervous system: dizziness, headache,

Psychological: euphoria, depression, nocturnal unrest, hallucinations, psychosis.

Endocrine: gynaecomastia.

Urogenital: impotence, incontinence of urine, retrograde ejaculation in men, failure of orgasm in women.

Skin: rash.

CHEM NAME	TRADE NAME	FORMULATION
clonidine	CATAPRES	0.1mg, 0.3mg
0.05–0.1mg three times daily.		
	CATAPRES PERLONGETS	0.25mg sustained-release
1–3 daily.		

These two formulations of clonidine are not directly interchangeable as the PERLONGETS are a slow-release formulation.

VASODILATORS

There are many different examples of this group. They may dilate arteries, veins or both. They are used in hypertension and cardiac failure.

They are used with diuretics and betablockers when these have been insufficient on their own.

HYDRALAZINE

Catogory III drug.
  Also used in the treatment of cardiac failure.
Contraindications:
Rapid heart rate and certain unusual cardiac conditions.
Precautions:
Prolonged treatment over 6 months may precipitate a condition similar to systemic lupus erythematous with the appearance of joint pains, fever and a skin rash. It usually subsides when the drug is stopped.
In the case of long-term treatment especially at doses over 100mg daily then 6 monthly urinalysis and testing for antinuclear factor should be performed. Also the acetylator status of the patient should be determined for these patients. This gives an indication of the speed at which the body metabolises substances.
Caution in cases of coronary artery disease (may worsen angina pectoris) or cerebrovascular disease.
Effects:
Systemic lupus erythematosus-like syndrome.
General: fever.
Cardiovascular: rapid heart rate, palpitations, fluid retention, aggravation of angina pectoris.
Respiratory: pleuritic chest pain.
Gastrointestinal: anorexia, nausea, vomiting, diarrhoea, hepatitis, obstructive jaundice.
Central nervous system: throbbing headache, dizziness, peripheral neuritis leading to parasthesiae.
Psychological: anxiety, depression.
Urogenital: kidney damage, impotence.
Blood disorders (necessitates drug withdrawal): changes in blood count, pancytopenia.
Skin: flushing, rashes.
Special senses: nasal congestion.

CHEM NAME	TRADE NAME	FORMULATION
hydralazine	APRESOLINE	25mg, 50mg

Hypertension: 25mg two or three times daily. Maximum 200mg daily.
Cardiac failure: 25mg two or three times daily. Maximum 50–75mg three or four times daily.

diazoxide	EUDEMINE	50mg

400–1000mg daily.

MINOXIDIL

Category III drug. This is only used in cases of severe hypertension when other treatment has failed.

Precautions:
Overgrowth of hair occurs in most patients and they should be specifically warned of this before treatment begins. Most revert to the pre-treatment state within 1–3 months after stopping the drug. Pericardial effusion may be produced and all patients should be regularly examined to exclude this development.

Effects:
Cardiovascular: oedema, rapid heart rate which may precipitate angina pectoris, palpitations, ECG changes.
Gastrointestinal: nausea.
Endocrine: breast tenderness.
Skin: overgrowth of hair.
Special senses: impaired hearing.

CHEM NAME	TRADE NAME	FORMULATION
minoxidil	LONITEN	2.5mg, 5mg, 10mg

Hypertension: 5mg daily increased as required. Maximum 50mg daily.

ALPHABLOCKERS

There are several types in this group.

PRAZOSIN

Cateogry III drug.
   This is related to the drugs CARDURA and HYTRIN. It is also used in the treatment of cardiac failure.

Precautions:
Some patients may react by producing a very low blood pressure as evidenced by dizziness, weakness or even loss of consciousness.

Effects:
These are seen in up to 60% of patients.
General: drowsiness, lack of energy, weakness, faintness, temporary loss of consciousness, fever, joint pains.
Cardiovascular: palpitations, postural hypotension, oedema,

breathlessness, rapid heart rate, angina pectoris, myocardial infarction.

Gastrointestinal: anorexia, dry mouth, nausea, vomiting, diarrhoea, constipation, abdominal discomfort and/or pain, liver function abnormalities, pancreatitis.

Central nervous system: dizziness, headache, vertigo, parasthesiae.

Psychological: nervousness, hallucinations, depression, mood changes, confusion, bad dreams.

Urogenital: frequency, impotence, incontinence, priapism.

Skin: rash, itching, alopecia, sweating.

Special senses: blurred vision, epistaxis, tinnitus, nasal congestion.

CHEM NAME	TRADE NAME	FORMULATION
doxazosin	CARDURA	1mg, 2mg, 4mg
Hypertension: 2–4mg daily. Maximum 16mg daily.		
prazosin	HYPOVASE	500mcg, 1mg, 2mg, 5mg
Hypertension: 1mg two or three times daily. Maximum 20mg daily.		
Cardiac failure: 4–20mg daily.		
terazosin	HYTRIN	1mg, 2mg, 5mg, 10mg
Hypertension: maintenance 2–10mg daily.		

INDORAMIN

Category III drug.
Contraindications:
Cardiac failure and those who are taking MAOI.
Precautions:
Renal or hepatic insufficiency, those with Parkinson's disease, epilepsy, depression or a history of depression and the elderly.
Effects:
These are seen in 30% of patients.
General: sedation.
Cardiovascular: palpitations.
Gastrointestinal: dry mouth, weight gain, increased appetite, constipation.
Central nervous system: headache, dizziness, Parkinson-like symptoms.
Psychological: depression, vivid dreams, sleep disturbance.
Gastrointestinal: dry mouth, weight gain.

Urogenital: failure of ejaculation.
Special senses: nasal congestion.

CHEM NAME	TRADE NAME	FORMULATION
indoramin	BARATOL	25mg, 50mg

Hypertension: 25mg twice daily. Maximum 200mg daily.

CALCIUM ANTAGONISTS

Category III drug.
Some of these are also commonly used in the treatment of angina pectoris.
They are relatively new and so many effects are probably not known. There are several groups of calcium anagonists whose effects vary somewhat. Simply stated there are two main groups:

- Type I which affect mainly blood vessels and include amlodipine, isradipine, nifedipine and nicardipine.
- Type II which mainly affect myocardium and include verapamil and diltiazem.

Sudden withdrawal may result in myocardial infarction.

TYPE I

The newer types such as amlodipine and isradipine seem to have less severe effects than nifedipine.
Precautions:
Care must be exercised in those with renal or hepatic impairment, some cases of cardiac arrythmias. It is not to be used in pregnant women and those who may become pregnant must use an effective form of contraception.
Hypotension or cardiac failure may be precipitated.
Effects:
General: tiredness.
Cardiovascular: oedema, palpitations, pain of the anginal type (nifedipine), cold extremities.
Central nervous system: headache, dizziness.
Gastrointestinal: jaundice, nausea, vomiting.
Skin: flushing, rash.

CHEM NAME	TRADE NAME	FORMULATION
amlodipine	ISTIN	5mg, 10mg

Hypertension and angina: 5–10mg daily.

isradipine	PRESCAL	2.5mg

Hypertension: 2–4 daily. Maximum 8 daily.

nicardipine	CARDENE	20mg, 30mg

Hypertension and angina: maintenance usually 30mg or 40mg twice daily.
Maximum 120mg daily.

nifedipine	ADALAT RETARD	10mg, 20mg

Hypertension: usually 10–40mg twice daily.

	ADALAT	5mg, 10mg

Angina: usually 5–20mg three times daily.
Raynaud's phenomenon: 10mg three times daily. Maximum 20mg three times daily.

	CALCILAT	10 mg

TYPE II

Contraindications:
They must not be used in those with untreated cardiac failure or in certain cardiac arrhythmias.
Precautions:
When used with betablockers there may be increased effects on cardiac function. Cardiac failure may be precipitated or worsened.
Effects:
Cardiovascular: flushing.
Gastrointestinal: nausea, vomiting, constipation.
Allergic reactions.

CHEM NAME	TRADE NAME	FORMULATION
diltiazem	ADIZEM	60mg
	ANGIOZEM	60mg
	BRITIAZEM	60mg
	TILDIEM	60mg

Angina: 3 daily. Increased to 6 daily if required.
Elderly: 2 daily initially.
Not for children.

	ADIZEM-SR	120mg continuous release

Angina: 2 daily. Increased to 4 daily if required.

Not for elderly or children.

verapamil	BERKATENS	40mg, 80mg, 120mg, 160mg
	CORDILOX	40mg, 80mg, 120mg, 160mg
	CORDILOX 160	160mg
	SECURON	120mg, 160mg

Hypertension: 80–160mg three times daily. Maximum 480mg daily.
Angina: 120mg three times daily.

	SECURON SR	240mg sustained-release
	UNIVER	120mg, 180mg, 240mg sustained-release

240mg daily; maximum 480mg daily.

THE RAUWOLFIA ALKALOIDS

Category III drug.
They are not commonly used these days because of their toxicity. They are widely used in Germany which serves to illustrate the differing practices in other countries.
Contraindications:
Depression, active peptic ulcer or ulcerative colitis.
Precautions:
Arrhythmias, myocardial infarction, pregnancy, lactation, bronchitis and asthma.
Cardiac failure may be precipitated.
Effects:
General: lethargy, drowsiness.
Cardiovascular: hypotension, slow pulse rate.
Gastrointestinal: diarrhoea, peptic ulceration, increased salivation.
Central nervous system: Parkinson-like symptoms.
Psychological: depression, confusion, bizarre dreams.
Urogenital: impairment of ejaculation.
Endocrine: galactorrhoea, gynaecomastia.
Skin: rash.
Special senses: nasal congestion.

CHEM NAME	TRADE NAME	FORMULATION
methoserpidine	DECASERPYL	5mg, 10mg

5–10mg daily. Maximum 50mg daily.

reserpine	SERPASIL	0.1mg, 0.25mg

Maintenance, up to 0.5mg daily.

COMMENTS.

Drugs are commonly used in the treatment of high blood pressure although there are efforts in a few areas to use relaxation or biofeedback techniques. However, the majority of patients seen in clinic will be taking one or more types of drugs.

In general, diuretics are prescribed first followed by a specific hypotensive agent such as a betablocker if control is insufficient.

There is a small group of people with so-called 'malignant' hypertension which is very severe and requires high doses of drugs. These cases should be treated in conjunction with medical advice as stopping or withdrawal of the drug may lead to serious consequences.

The majority of patients with hypertension can be approached with care. The diagnosis of hypertension is made on the basis of the level of the blood pressure and this is considered to vary with age.

The upper limits of normal are:

120/90 at age 20
160/95 at age 50
170/105 at age 75 ([8])

These levels are very much open to interpretation by doctors and some treat patients for hypertension when the blood pressure is as low as 160/90 even in middle-aged patients. There is no generally accepted norm and the practice in the UK differs from that in the rest of Europe.

As alternative practitioners, blood pressure is only one factor to be taken into account in diagnosis and treatment. I would be careful not to get obsessed with a particular set of figures. The overall picture is the important one.

Having said that, a blood pressure level which is not more than 20 or 30mm above each of the figures above taking into account the patient's age is OK to work with. For example, in a man of 50 if the blood pressure rises to 180/110 I would feel happy about continuing assuming that treatment was underway and effective. People are concerned about 'strokes' and cardiac conditions but levels of blood pressure have to be high for a long time. Sudden problems are not likely given the proviso of the above.

Always wait for an improvement before reducing the drugs and expect a rebound rise in blood pressure whenever the dose is lessened as well as perhaps the appearance of symptoms such as lightheadedness, dizziness and headache. Patients soon start to feel better, partly as a result of the treatment and partly as the drug effects lessen with the reduced dose. Adverse effects are experienced in around 70% of patients who take hypotensive agents.

Table of drug severities in increasing order of strength:

CATEGORY II
diuretics — medium potency
diuretics — high potency
methyldopa
CATEGORY III
clonidine
calcium antagonist, ACE inhibitor, betablockers
vasodilators
Rauwolfia alkaloid

Begin with the most powerful drug first. DO NOT STOP ANY HYPOTENSIVES SUDDENLY as cardiac problems may occur. This is particularly true of betablockers, calcium antagonists and clonidine. Once the hypotensive drug has been stopped move on to the diuretic.

Often the patient improves, the drugs are withdrawn and they have an improved level of health but with occasional flareups resulting from perhaps stressful events at home or work. It is not necessary for the patient to resort to drugs on each occasion. Relaxation, massage and specific treatment can all be used to help. As stated above, a short term elevated blood pressure is not going to kill people and it is possible to deal with these situations in other ways.

CASE

This is a more detailed analysis of the case which appeared in Chapter 3.

A woman of 83 years who had been treated for hypertension over the past 3 years. When she was originally diagnosed by her GP (on the basis of one blood pressure reading) she was started on ALDOMET 250mg three times daily. After only one dose she got up in the night to go to the toilet, fainted due to low blood pressure and did not regain full consciousness until some three days later. Her blood pressure in hospital showed that it fluctuated over a wide range.

On discharge she was stabilised on betablockers.

At the time of consultation currently her problems were tiredness (falling asleep every afternoon for several hours), poor memory, lack of concentration and poor appetite. Her blood pressure was 150/75.

She had an episode of dizziness six months previously for which she was prescribed STEMETIL.

Medication:

> TENORMIN LS 50mg three daily.
> bendrofluazide 5mg daily.
> STEMETIL 5mg three times daily.
> paracetamol 500mg two twice daily.

First check out each drug in turn.

TENORMIN LS is a betablocker used to treat hypertension, maximum dose is 100mg daily — this woman is being given 150mg daily.

Bendrofluazide is a diuretic used in conjunction with the betablocker for hypertension.

STEMETIL is usually used for nausea and vomiting but here for dizziness and loss of balance.

Paracetamol is an analgesic and was taken for a painful scar left by a chest operation many years before.

Looking at the side-effects of the drugs, particularly the TENORMIN LS and STEMETIL it can be seen that sedation is common. In view of the large dose of TENORMIN LS which is higher than that recommended it may be that most of this woman's symptoms are due to the drugs.

Her blood pressure was, in fact, low taking into account her age.

I stopped the STEMETIL first since that was for a short-term problem no longer present. She was irritable and anxious for several days as would be expected from the removal of a sedative. This settled and she soon felt more alert, no more sleeping in the day and her mental faculties became sharper.

Then the TENORMIN LS was reduced to two daily (100mg in all). Her blood pressure rose to 180/100 which was still satisfactory in view of her age and stabilised at 170/90.

After a short period of treatment again her TENORMIN LS

was reduced to one daily. The blood pressure rose to 190/110 and became stable at 180/100. She felt well with none of her presenting symptoms remaining.

Treatment continued and it may be in the future that her medication may be able to be reduced further. However, her diet was not amenable to change and in view of her age it may be that this was as far as things could be taken.

It is evident that her medication was a major factor in her symptomatology and once it had been reduced she felt better. At this age with degeneration of the cardiovascular system and atherosclerosis a certain level of blood pressure is required to supply blood to the vital organs. With conventional medical treatment and reduction of the blood pressure many symptoms are due to starving the brain of blood. Once the drugs and therefore their effects were lessened and her blood pressure became more 'normal' for her age she felt much better.

Diuretics

These are all Category II drugs unless they are used in severe cardiac or renal failure when Category V would be more appropriate. In these cases the high potency diuretics are used.

They are commonly used to treat oedema and fluid retention. This may be due to a discrete disease such as cardiac failure, a more symptomatic approach as in premenstrual fluid retention or oedema of unknown origin in some apparently fit women of child-bearing age.

They are also used either alone or with hypotensive agents to treat hypertension.

Potassium chloride is added to several diuretics especially the potent loop diuretics as potassium loss may develop as fluid is excreted from the body.

The symptoms of potassium deficiency, which is very difficult to diagnose biochemically until gross levels are attained, include apathy, confusion, drowsiness, polyuria, thirst, abdominal distension and muscle weakness.

CARBONIC ANHYDRASE INHIBITOR

Category II when used in oedema. Category III if used in epilepsy.

This is not commonly used now as a diuretic. It may also be used for epilepsy or as drops in cases of glaucoma.

CHEM NAME	TRADE NAME	FORMULATION
acetazolamide	DIAMOX	250mg

Initially 250–375mg once daily in the morning or on alternate days.
In premenstrual tension 125–375mg as single daily dose beginning 5–10 days before menstruation.

POTASSIUM SPARING DIURETICS

Category II drugs.
This group is considered to be of low potency (when compared with the others available) and so not to lead to loss of potassium. They are often combined with diuretics from the other groups so that potassium loss in those is minimised.
Potassium supplements should not be taken nor a potassium-rich diet. They are given for often severe oedema such as that seen with cardiac failure, hepatic failure and in cases of refractory oedema.

AMILORIDE

Category II drug.
Contraindications:
Those who take potassium supplements, cases of renal failure, severe progressive renal disease and diabetic renal disease.
Precautions:
In diabetic patients renal function must be determined before treatment begins.
Regular checks should be made on potassium levels since potassium conservation may occur. High potassium levels lead to lethargy, confusion, muscle weakness, irregular slow pulse and cardiac arrest eventually.
Patients with liver disease are more likely to develop side-effects from therapy.
Effects:
General: weakness, fatigue, back pain, neck and shoulder ache, pain in the extremities.
Cardiovascular: chest pain and angina pectoris, low blood pressure, palpitations.

Central nervous system: headache, dizziness, vertigo, paraesthesiae, tremors, tinnitus.
Psychological: nervousness, mental confusion, insomnia, depression, sleepiness.
Respiratory: cough, breathlessness.
Gastrointestinal: anorexia, nausea, vomiting, diarrhoea, constipation, abdominal pain, gastrointestinal bleeding, jaundice, thirst, dyspepsia, flatulence, peptic ulcer, liver function abnormalities.
Urogenital: impotence, decreased libido, polyuria, dysuria, bladder spasms, frequency of micturition.
Blood disorders: low white cell count, aplastic anaemia, eosinophilia.
Skin: itching, rash, dryness of mouth, alopecia.
Special senses: nasal congestion, visual disturbances.

CHEM NAME	TRADE NAME	FORMULATION
amiloride	AMILOSPARE	
	BERKAMIL	5mg
	MIDAMOR	5mg
1–4 daily.		
	AMILCO	5mg with 50mg hydrochlorothiazide
	VASETIC	5mg with 50mg hydrochlorothiazide

1–2 daily. Maximum 4 daily.
With the addition of a thiazide diuretic.

	FRUMIL	5mg with 40mg frusemide

1–2 daily.
With the addition of a high potency diuretic.

	FRUMIL LS	2.5mg with 20mg frusemide

Elderly: 1 daily.
With the addition of a high potency diuretic

	HYPERTANE	5mg with 50mg hydrochlorothiazide

1–2 daily. Maximum 4 daily.
With the addition of a thiazide diuretic.

	LASORIDE	5mg with 40mg frusemide

1–2 in the morning.
Elderly: adjust the dose according to renal function, response and serum electrolytes.
With the addition of a high potency diuretic.

	MODURET-25	2.5mg with 25mg

1–4 daily.
With the addition of a thiazide diuretic.

	hydrochlorothiazide
MODURETIC	5mg with 50mg hydrochlorothiazide
NORMETIC	5mg with 50mg hydrochlorothiazide

1–2 daily. Maximum of 4 daily.
With the addition of a thiazide diuretic.

SPIRONOLACTONE

Category II drug.
Contraindications:
Anuria, renal failure, progressive impairment of renal function
and Addison's disease.
Precautions:
There is some evidence that this drug may lead to the develop-
ment of carcinoma and this should be borne in mind before
treatment begins. Fluid and electrolyte balance should be
monitored periodically especially in the elderly and those with
renal or hepatic impairment. Potassium levels may rise to cause
death. Combining potassium supplements with spironolactone
is tantamount to medical negligence.
Effects:
General: drowsiness, lethargy.
Gastrointestinal: nausea, vomiting, hepatitis.
Central nervous system: headache, ataxia.
Psychological: mental confusion.
Endocrine: gynaecomastia (may be irreversible), menstrual
irregularities, masculinisation, deepening of voice in women,
breast enlargement and soreness.
Urogenital: loss of libido in men, impotence, oligospermia.
Skin: rashes.

CHEM NAME	TRADE NAME	FORMULATION
spironolactone	ALDACTONE	25mg, 50mg, 100mg
	DIATENSEC	50mg
	LARACTONE	25mg, 50mg, 100mg
	SPIRETIC	25mg, 100mg
	SPIROCTAN	25mg, 50mg
	SPIROLONE	25mg, 50mg, 100mg

Congestive cardiac failure: maintenance 75–200mg daily.

SPIROSPARE
LASILACTONE   50mg with 20mg
                     frusemide

1–4 daily.
With the addition of a high potency diuretic.

TRIAMTERENE

Category II drug.
Contraindications:
Renal failure.
Precautions:
Hepatic or renal insufficiency, those predisposed to gout and with hypotensive agents (further lowering of blood pressure occurs).
Blood urea and serum electrolytes should be monitored periodically.
Effects:
General: weakness.
Cardiovascular: low blood pressure
Gastrointestinal: nausea, vomiting, diarrhoea, dry mouth.
Central nervous system: headache.
Urogenital: renal failure.
Allergy: anaphylaxis.
Blood disorders: thrombocytopenia, anaemia.
Skin: rash, photosensitivity.

CHEM NAME	TRADE NAME	FORMULATION
triamterene	DYTAC	50mg

3–5 daily, alternate day therapy recommended after one week.

THIAZIDE DIURETIC

Category II drug.
These are medium potency diuretics and are widely used for the treatment of oedema and hypertension either alone or with other drugs.
Contraindications:
Anuria, severe renal and hepatic failure. Diuretics should not be given at the same time as lithium salts.

Precautions:
All the thiazides may precipitate or aggravate diabetes mellitus and gout.
Elderly patients should be closely monitored.
Caution with renal and hepatic dysfunction. Renal function should be monitored in these patients.
Effects:
General: worsening of gout.
Respiratory: pulmonary oedema with allergic pneumonitis.
Gastrointestinal: nausea, vomiting, pancreatitis.
Central nervous system: dizziness, transient ischaemic attacks.
Endocrine: worsening or development of diabetes mellitus.
Urogenital: impotence especially with bendrofluazide.
Blood: thrombocytopenia, haemolytic anaemia, granulocytopenia, agranulocytosis.
Skin: rashes with photosensitivity.
Special senses: worsening of myopia.

CHEM NAME	TRADE NAME	FORMULATION
bendrofluazide	APRINOX	2.5mg, 5mg
	BERKOZIDE	2.5mg, 5mg
	CENTYL	2.5mg, 5mg
	NEO-NACLEX	5mg

Maintenance: there is a difference of opinion amongst manufacturers here. Some quote 5–10mg once or twice weekly, others 2.5–10mg daily.
Hypertension, 2.5–5mg once daily.
Cardiac failure 5–10mg daily or on alternate days.

	CENTYL K	2.5mg with potassium chloride 573mg
	NEO-NACLEX K	2.5mg with potassium chloride 630mg

Maintenance 1–4 daily or on alternate days.
With the addition of a potassium supplement.

	TENAVOID	3mg with meprobamate 200mg

Indicated for premenstrual syndrome.
1 three times daily beginning 5–7 days before the expected onset of the next period.
Controlled drug.
With the addition of a tranquilliser.

benzthiazide	DYTIDE	25mg with 50mg triamterene

Maintenance 1–2 alternate days.
With the addition of a low potency diuretic.

chlorothiazide	SALURIC	500mg

Oedema, 1 or 2 once or twice daily or intermittently. Hypertension, 1 or 2 daily in single or divided doses. Maximum 4 daily.

chlorthalidone	HYGROTON	50mg, 100mg

Oedema: maintenance 100mg twice weekly.
Hypertension 25–50mg daily.

	HYGROTON K	25mg with potassium chloride 500mg

Hypertension, 1 or 2 daily.
Oedema, 1 or 2 daily or 2–4 three times a week.

	KALSPARE	50mg with 50mg triamterene

1–2 daily.
With the addition of a low potency diuretic.
Not a thiazide but the same comments apply.

cyclo-penthiazide	NAVIDREX	0.5mg

0.25–1mg daily. Maximum 1.5mg daily.

	NAVIDREX K	0.25mg with potassium chloride 600mg

1–4 daily. Maximum 6 daily.
With the addition of a potassium supplement.

	NAVISPARE	0.25mg with 2.5mg amiloride

1–2 daily.
With the addition of a low potency diuretic.

hydro-chlorothiazide	ESIDREX	25mg, 50mg
	HYDROSALURIC	25mg, 50mg

Maintenance 25–50mg on alternate days.

	DYAZIDE	25mg with 50mg triamterene
	TRIAMCO	25mg with 50mg triamterene

Hypertension, initially 1 daily.
Oedema, 1 daily or 2 on alternate days. Maximum 4 daily. With the addition of a low potency diuretic.

mefruside	BAYCARON	25mg

Maximum 4 daily in oedema. Maintenance, 1 daily or on alternate days.
Not a thiazide but the same comments apply.

methy-clothiazide	ENDURON	5mg

2.5–5mg daily; maximum 10mg daily.

metolazone	METENIX	5mg

Hypertension, 5mg on alternate days.

Oedema: 5–10mg daily as single dose. Maximum 80mg in 24 hours.
Not a thiazide but the same comments apply. This drug has a greater
effect on the blood sugar.

hydro- flumethazide	HYDRENOX	50mg

Oedema, maintenance, 25–50mg on alternate days.
Hypertension, 25–50mg daily.

	ALDACTIDE 50	50mg with 50mg spironolactone
	ALDACTIDE 25	25mg with 25mg spironolactone

1 to 8 ALDACTIDE 25 or 4 ALDACTIDE 50 daily.
With the addition of a low potency diuretic.

polythiazide	NEPHRIL	1mg

1–4 daily.

NON-THIAZIDE DIURETIC

Category II drug.
Precautions.
Renal or hepatic impairment.
These drugs may cause severely low potassium levels which
may induce serious ventricular arrhythmias. Symptoms would
include palpitations with fainting.
Effects:
General: tiredness, muscle weakness.
Central nervous system: headache.
Gastrointestinal: nausea.

CHEM NAME	TRADE NAME	FORMULATION
indapamide	NATRILIX	2.5mg
1 daily.		
xipamide	DIUREXAN	20mg

Hypertension, 1–2 daily.
Oedema, 1–4 daily.

LOOP DIURETIC (HIGH POTENCY)

These are often in Category II but may be considered to be in
Category V when used for severe lifethreatening disease such
as severe cardiac failure or renal failure.
These are the potent diuretics used for severe cases of oedema

as seen in cardiac failure. They produce a marked diuresis and for this reason are usually taken in the morning. They can precipitate urinary retention in patients with some degree of prostatic enlargement because of the large increase in urinary excretion. Since they are so powerful potassium depletion occurs very easily and most are given with potassium supplements either as an integral part of the tablet or as extra medication.

BUMETANIDE

Category II or V (see above).
Contraindications:
Hepatic coma and special care taken in cases of severe electrolyte depletion.
As with all diuretics it should not be given at the same as lithium salts.
Precautions:
Excessive removal of oedema especially in the elderly may precipitate marked changes in the cardiovascular system with circulatory collapse. Regular checks of serum electrolytes should be made.
Care should be taken when prescribed to patients who take hypotensive agents.
Periodic checks on urine and blood sugar should be made in diabetics and those suspected of latent diabetes.
Effects:
These are very similar to those of frusemide (see below) although the following are those listed in the literature.
General: muscular cramps in the legs.
Gastrointestinal: abdominal discomfort.
Endocrine: gynaecomastia.
Blood disorders: thrombocytopenia.
Skin: rashes.

CHEM NAME	TRADE NAME	FORMULATION
bumetanide	BURINEX	1mg, 5mg

Usually 1mg daily adjusted according to patient's response.

	TRADE NAME	FORMULATION
	BURINEX K	0.5mg with potassium chloride 573mg

1–4 daily.
With the addition of a potassium supplement.

ETHACRYNIC ACID

Category V.
This drug is extremely powerful and is only used in severe cases of oedema.
Precautions:
Those with advanced liver cirrhosis. This drug may precipitate hepatic coma and death in such patients.
Patients should be weighed regularly throughout treatment. There should also be regular checks of serum electrolyte and blood urea levels.
In the elderly there is a risk of concentration of blood due to extreme diuresis leading to the possibility of strokes or pulmonary embolism.
Effects:
Acute gout may be precipitated.
General: fever, shivering, fatigue.
Gastrointestinal: anorexia, malaise, abdominal discomfort or pain, dysphagia, nausea, vomiting, diarrhoea, gastrointestinal bleeding, jaundice, acute pancreatitis.
The onset of profuse watery diarrhoea is an indication for stopping the drug.
Central nervous system: headache, tinnitus, vertigo.
Psychological: apprehension, confusion.
Urogenital: haematuria.
Blood disorders: neutropenia, agranulocytosis, thrombocytopenia.
Special senses: blurred vision, deafness (usually reversible but permanent in some).
Skin: purpura, rashes.

CHEM NAME	TRADE NAME	FORMULATION
ethacrynic acid	EDECRIN	50mg

Minimum effective dose usually 1–3 daily. Maximum 8 daily.

FRUSEMIDE

Category II or V (see above).
Contraindications:
Anuria, electrolyte deficiency and pre-comatose states associated with liver cirrhosis and sulphonamide sensitivity.

Precautions:
The side-effects of antibiotics affecting the kidney may be increased. Diabetes mellitus may be aggravated or precipitated by this drug. Care should be taken when hypotensive agents are also prescribed.
Patients with urinary problems or prostatic hypertrophy have an increased risk of developing urinary retention.
Gout may be precipitated.

Effects:
General: malaise, drowsiness. Raised uric acid levels which may precipitate an attack of gout.
Cardiovascular: postural hypotension, fainting.
Gastrointestinal: nausea, vomiting, gastric upset, diarrhoea, jaundice.
Psychological: reduced mental alertness.
Endocrine: raised blood sugar.
Urogenital: excess urination, dehydration.
Blood disorders: agranulocytosis, thrombocytopenia, haemolytic anaemia.
Skin: rashes.
Special senses: tinnitus, vertigo, deafness especially with high doses. There is evidence of high tone deafness in over 6% of patients.
Visual disturbances.

CHEM NAME	TRADE NAME	FORMULATION
frusemide	ALUZINE	20mg, 40mg
	DRYPTAL	40mg
	FRUMAX	
	FRUSID	40mg
	LASIX	20mg, 40mg
	RUSYDE	
20–80mg daily or on alternate days.		
	DIUMIDE-K CONTINUS	40mg with potassium chloride 600mg
1 daily.		
	FRUSENE	40mg with 50mg triamterene
½–2 daily.		
With the addition of a low potency diuretic.		
	LASIKAL	20mg with potassium chloride 750mg
1–4 daily.		
	LASIX+K	40mg with potassium

chloride 750mg
as separate tablets
1 tablet of frusemide in the morning and 1 tablet of potassium chloride
at noon and evening.

PIRETANIDE

Category II or V (see above).
This is a very similar drug to frusemide (see above).
Contraindications:
Severe electrolyte disturbances.
Precautions:
People with urinary problems or prostatic hypertrophy have an
increased risk of developing urinary retention.
Toxicity of some antibiotics may be increased — cephalospor-
ins and the kidney, aminoglycosides and the ear.
Potassium depletion may occur. Severe hepatic disease may
develop into coma if this drug is used.
Diuretics may precipitate or aggravate diabetes mellitus.
Serum electrolytes should be regularly monitored in patients
with severe impaired renal function, severe liver cirrhosis,
those liable to develop electrolyte imbalance, where digoxin or
corticosteroids are given.
Effects:
General: muscle cramps.
Gastrointestinal: nausea, vomiting, diarrhoea.
Skin: rashes.

CHEM NAME	TRADE NAME	FORMULATION
piretanide 1 or 2 daily.	ARELIX	6mg

COMMENTS

Diuretics are used for a wide range of disorders where oedema
is a symptom. These include cardiac failure, renal disease,
premenstrual tension, oedema of unknown origin (according to
Western medicine) or in hypertension. Clearly some conditions
are more serious than others and so it is helpful to try and
discover the original condition requiring medication.

Table of drug strength in order of increasing strength:

CATEGORY II
- low potency
- medium potency (mainly the thiazides)

CATEGORY II or V
- high potency:
  frusemide
  piretanide
  bumetanide

CATEGORY V
- high potency:
  ethacrynic acid

High potency diuretics are used in the severe forms of oedema of cardiac and renal disease. As diuretics remove water they chiefly affect the kidney and lead to problems of thirst, polyuria and tiredness. Potassium is also lost along with the water and potassium deficiency is not uncommon. In fact it is probably more widespread than is generally realised. Potassium loss is more marked with the more powerful drugs and so potassium supplements are usually given with the diuretics. With many thiazide prescriptions potassium is not routinely given. Potassium deficiency leads to symptoms of . . . thirst, polyuria and tiredness!

Withdrawal leads to the reappearance of oedema and scanty urination. It may be possible for patients to take the diuretic on a symptomatic basis for a while, e.g. every 2–3 days when the oedema builds up. This is more likely to be possible in mild cases rather than cardiac failure.

With more severe disease then more care has to be taken since any increase in oedema, e.g. of the pulmonary type is accompanied by more severe symptoms.

Cardiac Failure

This is a disease of the cardiovascular system characterised by oedema. The site of the oedema depends on which part of the heart has the predominant problem. So left ventricular failure leads to pulmonary oedema and right ventricular failure leads to systemic oedema. In practice however mixed types are usually seen. This condition is clearly serious in terms of manifestations and origin and so must be approached with care. The drugs often used are consequently very powerful in their actions.

CARDIAC GLYCOSIDE

Category III drug.

This is derived from the foxglove plant and is an example of a drug which has been developed from herbal uses.

It is one of only very few drugs currently available which will lead to an increase in the strength of contraction of the heart.

Contraindications:

Certain cases of abnormal heart rhythm.

Digitalis toxicity is commonly seen because the effective dose is very similar to the toxic dose. Around 30% of patients have such toxicity and of those affected the mortality rate is 4–36% depending upon the particular problem produced.

Precautions:

Intoxication with this drug may produce abnormal heart rhythms of the type for which it was first prescribed.

Low potassium levels increase sensitivity to the drug and care should be taken if diuretics, corticosteroids or carbenoxolone are prescribed concurrently.

Effects:

General: drowsiness, fatigue, malaise.

Cardiovascular: palpitations, irregular heart rates of many types (some are fatal), heart failure.

Gastrointestinal: salivation, nausea, vomiting, anorexia, diarrhoea, abdominal pain.

Central nervous system: headache, facial pain, aphasia, dizziness, EEG changes, epilepsy.Psychological: depression, nervousness, agitation, restlessness, amnesia, bad dreams, mental confusion, disorientation, delirium, hallucinations (may herald the onset of toxicity), acute psychosis.

Endocrine: gynaecomastia, breast enlargement in women.

Blood disorders: thrombocytopenia, eosinophilia..

Skin: sweating, rash, itching.

Special senses: objects appear yellow or green (less commonly red, brown, blue or white).

Checking the serum levels of the drug can give an indication as to whether digoxin toxicity is occurring but this is by no means infallible. Toxicity can still occur where blood levels are fairly low.

CHEM NAME	TRADE NAME	FORMULATION
digoxin	LANOXIN	0.25mg
	LANOXIN 125	0.125mg
	LANOXIN-PG	62.5mcg
	LANOXIN-PG ELIXIR	50mcg/ml

Maintenance 0.25–0.5mg daily.
Elderly: maintenance 0.125–0.25mg daily.

lanatoside C	CEDILANID	0.25mg

Maintenance 1–6 daily.

XANTHINE

This group of drugs is used to treat wheezing and asthma. In this case it used in cases of pulmonary oedema where respiratory symptoms are present — see Chapter 8 for details.
Category V when used for pulmonary oedema — a manifestation of severe cardiac failure which can lead to distressing symptoms and signs.

CHEM NAME	TRADE NAME	FORMULATION
aminophylline	PECRAM	225mg

2 daily.

	PHYLLOCONTIN CONTINUS	100mg, 225mg sustained-release

2x225mg twice daily.

	PHYLLOCONTIN FORTE	350mg sustained-release

1–2 twice daily.

theophylline	UNIPHYLLIN CONTINUS	200mg, 300mg, 400mg

Less than 70Kg, 300mg twice daily. Over 70Kg, 400mg twice daily.

PARTIAL BETA1 AGONIST

Category V drug.
Precautions:
Acute cardiac failure.
The drug should be stopped in patients who deteriorate to the point where they become symptomatic at rest. If the drug is withdrawn, the patient should be carefully observed.

Caution with impaired renal function.
Effects:
General: muscle cramp.
Cardiovascular: angina and chest pain, palpitations.
Central nervous system: headache, dizziness.
Gastrointestinal complaints.
Skin: rash.

CHEM NAME	TRADE NAME	FORMULATION
xamoterol 1 twice daily.	CORWIN	200mg

COMMENTS

Table of drugs used in cardiac failure in order of increasing strength:

CATEGORY II
- diuretics:
  low potency
  medium potency

CATEGORY III
- digoxin
- ACE inhibitors
- vasodilators

CATEGORY V
- diuretic:
  high potency
- xanthine compounds
- xamoterol

Note 1: drugs which increase the force of cardiac contraction, namely digoxin and xamoterol, may be used for mild or severe cases. Check in each individual case.

Note 2: Occasionally drugs such as amiodarone (see Chapter 5) and xamoterol are used to treat severe ventricular arrhythmias. Again check in each case.

Vasodilators are of several types. Venodilators such as isosorbide dinitrate are used primarily for symptoms of oedema and congestion. Arteriolar dilators such as hydralazine are used primarily for symptoms of cold extremities and poor circulation. Prazosin is an example of a dilator of arteries and veins.

They lead to severe effects in many people and it is this which restricts their use.

Cardiac failure requiring this degree of medication is a serious condition and great care must be exercised in treatment. It may be advisable to seek medical advice before taking on such a case.

Angina Pectoris

Angina pectoris is a pain in the chest due to lack of blood supply to the heart muscle (ischaemic heart disease). There is an association with atherosclerosis. The conventional approach is to control the pain with drugs and if this medical approach fails to resort to coronary bypass surgery.

NITRATE

These are also used in the treatment of cardiac failure.

They can be used either symptomatically in which cases they fall into Category I or prophylactically when they must be put into Category III (although below betablockers which are much more powerful in their action).

There are several forms of nitrate available now. Some are taken for the symptomatic relief of pain at the time it happens and others are to be taken regularly. All have similar actions in dilating blood vessels. These effects are not confined to the heart.

When taken symptomatically patients are often told to take a tablet before exercise so that the pain does not appear and more exercise may be done. This is quite dangerous since the pain of angina is to prevent excessive exercise which the weakened heart muscle cannot deal with. If drugs are taken which allow more exercise then this may be harmful. It is better, if necessary to take nitrates after the pain has occurred. Even better to let the pain subside of its own accord with rest.

Withdrawal of the nitrates may lead to arterial spasm. This can manifest as pain of angina pectoris or myocardial infarction. Some patients may also experience lack of circulation to the extremities which may result in gangrene if severe.

Contraindications:

Acute myocardial infarction, acute circulatory failure, hypotension, marked anaemia, head trauma, cerebral haemorrhage.

Precautions:
These drugs may give rise to low blood pressure and fainting. The effects of alcohol may be increased and patients should be specifically warned of these problems.

Caution in hypothyroidism, hypothermia, malnutrition, severe liver and renal disease.

Effects on the cerebral circulation as a result of hypotension areprobably very common and it is wise in those with evidence of such problems to begin with a low dose.

Effects:
Cardiovascular: facial flushing, dizziness, lightheadedness, hypotension, rapid heart rate or very slow heart rate (both these effects may have serious consequences for those with severe atherosclerosis), coldness of the skin, weakness and other signs of reduced cerebral blood flow, peripheral oedema if used in left ventricular failure.

Gastrointestinal: nausea, vomiting, sublingual administration may give burning sensation on the tongue.

Central nervous system: throbbing headache, transient episodes of dizziness. Development of transient ischaemic attacks.

Blood: methaemoglobinaemia.

Skin: reddening of skin if administration is by skin patch.

CHEM NAME	TRADE NAME	FORMULATION
glyceryl	CORO-NITRO	0.4mg/dose (aerosol)
trinitrate	NITROLINGUAL	0.4mg/dose (aerosol)

1–2 doses at onset of attack or prior to exertion, maximum 3 doses per attack.

	DEPONIT	5mg, 10mg (adhesive patches)
	TRANSIDERM-NITRO	5mg, 10mg (adhesive patches)

Commence with 5mg patch and increase to 10mg if necessary.

	NITROCONTIN CONTINUS	2.6mg, 6.4mg sustained -release

2.6–6.4mg twice daily.

	PERCUTOL	2% ointment

Apply, without rubbing, 3–4 hourly or less frequently as required.

	SUSCARD BUCCAL	1mg, 2mg, 3mg, 5mg

Acute attacks, initially 1mg as required. Chronic cases, 1mg three times daily increasing strength and frequency if necessary.

Chronic heart failure, initially 5mg three times daily. Acute situations, 5mg repeated until symptoms abate.

	SUSTAC	2.6mg, 6.4mg, 10mg

sustained-release
2.6–12.8mg two or three times daily.

| isosorbide dinitrate | CEDOCARD RETARD | 20mg, 40mg sustained-release |
20–80mg twice daily.

CEDOCARD TABS.   5mg, 10mg, 20mg, 40mg
Acute attack, 5mg sublingually.
Prophylaxis, 5–40mg swallowed three or four times daily.
Cardiac failure: 10–40mg three or four times daily.

ISOKET RETARD   20mg, 40mg
                  sustained-release
20–40mg twice daily. Maximum 160mg daily.

ISORDIL   10mg, 30mg
40–120mg daily.
Cardiac failure: 10–60mg orally four times daily.

ISORDIL TEMBIDS   40mg sustained-release
1–3 daily.

ISORDIL
SUBLINGUAL   5mg
1 or 2 sublingually two or three hourly.

SONI-SLO   20mg, 40mg
             sustained-release
40–120mg daily.

SORBICHEW   5mg
1 or 2 chewed during an acute attack.

SORBID SA   20mg, 40mg
              sustained-release
20–80mg twice daily.

SORBITRATE   10mg, 20mg
10–40mg three or four times daily.

VASCARDIN   10mg, 30mg
Acute attack 5–10mg sublingually; prophylaxis 30–120mg daily.
Cardiac failure: 10–30mg three or four times daily.

| isosorbide mononitrate | ELANTAN | 10mg, 20mg, 40mg |
Maintenance 40–80mg daily. Maximum 120mg daily.
Cardiac failure: same dose.

ELANTAN LA   50mg sustained-release
One daily.

IMDUR   60mg sustained-release
1–2 daily.

ISMO   10mg, 20mg, 40mg
Maintenance, 20mg two or three times daily. Maximum 120mg daily.

Cardiac failure: maintenance 60mg daily. Maximum 120mg daily.

	ISOTRATE	20mg

Maintenance 1–6 daily.
Cardiac failure: 2–3 daily.

	MCR–50	50mg sustained-release

1–2 daily.

	MONIT	20mg
	MONIT LS	10mg

Maintenance 20mg two or three times daily.

	MONO-CEDOCARD	10mg, 20mg, 40mg

20–120mg daily.

pentaerythritol tetranitrate	CARDIACAP	30mg sustained-release

1 twice daily.

	MYCARDOL	30mg

2 three or four times daily.

COMMENTS

All the drugs used to treat angina pectoris are symptomatic, that
is, they are designed to stop pain. They make no attempt to
solve the underlying problem and, indeed, may make it worse
because they weaken the heart further.
Table of drugs listed in order of increasing strength:

CATEGORY I
- nitrates — symptomatic.
CATEGORY III
- nitrates — prophylactic
- betablockers, calcium antagonists

Surgery would clearly be a more severe form of treatment
than calcium antagonists or betablockers.
Sudden withdrawal, particularly of the more powerful drugs
may lead to severe anginal attacks or even coronary thrombosis.
Therefore, reduction must be gradual as treatment progresses.
Withdrawal will lead to an aggravation of the angina perhaps
with more pain or a decrease in exercise tolerance.

CASE

A man aged 51 presented for treatment with symptoms of
angina pectoris since a myocardial infarction 12 months previ-

ously. His exercise limit was walking 100–150 yards and this was reduced in cold weather.

Medication:

> glyceryl trinitrate 1mg when required.
> TENORMIN 100mg daily.
> ISMO 10mg three times daily.

Check on the drug details.

Glyceryl trinitrate is a nitrate to be taken symptomatically and ISMO a nitrate taken prophylactically. The dose of ISMO is low when compared with the usual maintenance.

TENORMIN is a betablocker taken regularly to slow the heart, reduce the amount of work it is capable of and so prevent attacks of angina.

In view of this amount of medication however the patient is still having great problems with only 100 yards of walking possible before he has to stop.

The first drug to begin with is the TENORMIN. After treatment had been proceeding for several weeks the patient began to improve with more exercise and less pain. He was able to walk further with little pain despite a cold winter. The TENORMIN was reduced to 50mg daily. He developed more pain for several weeks and noticed that he was able to only walk about 100 yards again. This is to be expected with a reduced dose of betablocker.

After each reduction further treatment followed and time was allowed for the case to stabilise.

Thus, after some 4 months he was having mild anginal attacks about once per week, his exercise limit was now several miles each day with use of an exercise bicycle at home also. He was no longer taking the nitrate for attacks but merely letting the pain subside by resting.

The ISMO was reduced in a similar fashion to the TENORMIN with reduction by 10mg each time — the middle of the day dosage removed first. The ISMO was stopped after 2 more months of treatment.

After 12 months of treatment the patient was on no medication, he was well with infrequent attacks of pain. His exercise level was good and he felt better than he had for many years.

Lipid (fat) reduction

These all fall into Category II unless given for severe familial hypercholesterolaemias in which case they will be in Category V.

This group of drugs is used to reduce the level of certain fats/fatty acids in the blood particularly cholesterol. It is believed that an increased level of these substances can lead to early and severe forms of ischaemic heart disease. Whilst this is certainly true for the rare forms of familial hyperlipidaemias there is little evidence to show that it is true for the vast majority of people with a raised cholesterol level. In fact there has been increasing evidence that a LOW cholesterol level may be associated with certain chronic disease states.

Before any patient embarks on drug treatment for raised levels of lipids there must be attempts to control other risk factors. These include smoking, use of alcohol, overweight, lack of exercise and other causes of raised levels such as diabetes mellitus, hypothyroidism.

Because these treatments tend to be long term there must be estimation on at least two occasions of lipid levels, blood count and liver function tests. Lipid levels must also be checked at regular intervals.

These drugs would seem to primarily affect the liver since in animal experiments high doses produce liver tumours. This has never been confirmed in humans but the tendency is there it seems.

I have listed the contraindications and effects of several drugs. Those which are not mentioned are similar particularly in terms of their gastrointestinal symptoms.

Clofibrate is the drug which has been studied most extensively over the years. The others are probably very similar in their effects. The problems seem to arise, not so much from short term effects, as from long term usage. Therefore a number of trials in which clofibrate was taken for several years has revealed a whole range of serious health risks. This is important to bear in mind given that patients are told to take these drugs for many years.

As to the effect on cardiac disease and mortality from such disease there is conflicting evidence.

ISOBUTYRIC ACID DERIVATIVE

CLOFIBRATE

The results of the long term multicentre WHO trial reveal that there is increased risk of tumours particularly of gastrointestinal or respiratory tract, deaths from respiratory infections, pyelonephritis, pancreatitis and peptic ulcer, gallstones requiring surgery, onset of diabetes mellitus.

Contraindications:
This must not be used in those with or a history of gallbladder disease or gallstones, renal or hepatic impairment.

Precautions:
Care must be exercised in those with low serum albumin levels eg nephrotic syndrome.
It may change the insulin requirements of those with diabetes mellitus.

Effects:
General: weakness, drowsiness, weight gain, lupus-like syndrome.
Cardiovascular: angina pectoris, intermittent claudication, pulmonary embolism (increases in these three seen in one drug trial). Cardiac arrhythmias, fluid retention.
Respiratory: Tumours. Pulmonary embolism.
Gastrointestinal: stomatitis, indigestion, nausea, diarrhoea, gallstones, pancreatitis (possible), changes in liver function tests.
Central nervous system: giddiness.
Urogenital: impotence.
Blood: rise in lipid levels, leucopenia, agranulocytosis, changes in haemoglobin levels.
Skin: appearance or worsening of xanthomata.

CHEM NAME	TRADE NAME	FORMULATION
clofibrate 20–30mg/Kg daily.	ATROMID S	500mg
fanofibrate Maintenance of 2–4 daily.	LIPANTIL	100mg

BEZAFIBRATE

Also see clofibrate.

Contraindications:
This must not be given to those with severe renal or hepatic impairment, nephrotic syndrome.
Effects:
General: tiredness.
Gastrointestinal: fullness of stomach, nausea, indigestion, abdominal pain necessitating stopping treatment in 1%, enlargement of liver.
Central nervous system: headache.
Urogenital: impotence

CHEM NAME	TRADE NAME	FORMULATION
bezafibrate 3 daily.	BEZALIP	200mg
1 daily.	BEZALIP-MONO	400mg

GEMFIBROZIL

Also see clofibrate.
Contraindications:
This must not be used in those with alcoholism, gallstones or hepatic impairment.
Precautions:
Care must be taken in those with renal impairment.
Effects:
General: painful extremities, muscle pains, joint pains. Infections such as common cold, cough and urinary tract affections are more common.
Gastrointestinal: dry mouth, abdominal pain, constipation, diarrhoea, nausea, epigastric pain, vomiting, flatulence.
Central nervous system: headache, dizziness, blurred vision, parasthesia, tinnitus, fainting.
Psychological: insomnia.
Urogenital: impotence.
Endocrine: hyperglycaemia.
Blood: leucopenia, low potassium levels.
Skin: rash, dermatitis, itching, urticaria.

CHEM NAME	TRADE NAME	FORMULATION
gemfibrozil	LOPID	300mg

NICOTINIC ACID DERIVATIVE

CHEM NAME	TRADE NAME	FORMULATION
acipimox	OLBETAM	250mg
2–3 daily. Maximum 1200 daily.		
nicofuranose	BRADILAN	250mg
2–4 three times daily.		

BILE ACID SEQUESTRANT

The main effects of these drugs are on the gastrointestinal system since they interfere with the absorption of factors within the bowel.

Effects:
Gastrointestinal: nausea, bloating, constipation (50%), anorexia, nausea, heartburn, diarrhoea, pancreatitis (possible), folic acid deficiency.
Blood: bleeding due to Vitamin K deficiency.
Bone: osteoporosis, osteomalacia.
Skin: rash, pruritus.

CHEM NAME	TRADE NAME	FORMULATION
cholestyramine	QUESTRAN	4G sachets
	QUESTRAN A	4G sachets
	(low sugar)	
3–6 sachets daily. Maximum 9 daily.		
colestipol	COLESTID	granules
5–30G daily.		

BUTYLPHENOL

Effects:
Cardiovascular: ECG changes.
Gastrointestinal: (lead to stopping treatment in about 3%) anorexia, diarrhoea, heartburn, abdominal pain, changes in liver function tests, gastrointestinal bleeding,.
Central nervous system: headache, dizziness, parasthesiae, tinnitus.
Psychological: insomnia.
Urogenital: impotence.

Endocrine: enlargement of goitre.
Blood: eosinophilia, increased in lipid levels, fall in haemoglobin levels, thrombocytopenia.
Skin: rash, pruritus.
Special senses: blurred vision, conjunctivitis.

CHEM NAME	TRADE NAME	FORMULATION
probucol
4 daily.	LURSELLE	250mg

MARINE TRIGLYCERIDES

This is a 'natural' substance rather than a drug and so very few problems are experienced.
Precautions:
Patients with bleeding disorders such as haemophilia or those receiving anticoagulants must be closely monitored.
Effects:
Gastrointestinal: belching, nausea.

CHEM NAME	TRADE NAME	FORMULATION
eicosa-
pentaenoic acid
5 capsules or 5ml twice daily.	MAXEPA	180mg with docosa-
hexaenoic acid

HMG CoA REDUCTASE INHIBITOR

This is a very new drug and there is little information available at present.
It is only used when there are very high levels of lipid in the blood or in those who do not respond to other treatments.
Contraindications:
This drug must not be used in those with hepatic disease or those taking the oral contraceptive.
Precautions:
Care must be taken with those who have a history of hepatic disease.
Liver function tests must be performed before treatment has begun and monitored during treatment.

Effects:
General: muscle pains and weakness, fatigue.
Gastrointestinal: constipation, diarrhoea, nausea, indigestion, flatulence.
Central nervous system: headache.
Skin: rash.

CHEM NAME	TRADE NAME	FORMULATION
simvastatin	ZOCOR	10mg, 20mg
Usually 10–40mg daily.		

Circulatory Disorders

Peripheral vascular disease such as Raynaud's phenomenon and periperhal atherosclerosis may be treated by drugs. These conditions are notoriously difficult to affect by any means other than stopping smoking and loss of excess weight. The use of drugs in such conditions is often useless and certainly not of great benefit in the remainder. There is no great faith in these drugs even in conventional circles. You may also see some of these drugs used in dementia due to degenerative arterial disease.

ANTIHISTAMINE

Category II.
  See Chapter 8 for details.

CHEM NAME	TRADE NAME	FORMULATION
cinnarizine	STUGERON FORTE	75mg
1 three times daily.		

CALCIUM OVERLOAD REGULATOR

Category II.
Precautions:
Care must be taken if prescribed in those with glaucoma.

Effects:
Gastrointestinal: nausea, heartburn.
Central nervous system: headache, tingling, dizziness.
Skin: flushing, sweating.

CHEM NAME	TRADE NAME	FORMULATION
cyclandelate	CYCLOBRAL	400mg
	CYCLOSPASMOL	400mg, 400mg/5ml
1 three or four times daily.		

NICOTINIC ACID DERIVATIVE

Category II drug.
Effects:
General: feelings of heat particularly in the upper part of the body, flushing.
Gastrointestinal: indigestion, diarrhoea, abdominal pain, activation of peptic ulcer, jaundice, changes in liver function.
Central nervous system: pounding headache.
Skin: pruritus, rash.
Special senses: blurring of vision.

CHEM NAME	TRADE NAME	FORMULATION
inositol	HEXOPAL	500mg, 1G/5ml
2 three or four times daily.		
	HEXOPAL FORTE	750mg
2 twice daily.		
nicofuranose	BRADILAN	250mg
2–4 three times daily.		
nicotinyl alcohol	RONICOL	25mg
1–2 four times daily.		
	RONICOL TIMESPAN	150mg
1–2 twice daily.		

PERIPHERAL AND CEREBRAL ACTIVATOR

Category II drug.

Effects:
Gastrointestinal: nausea, epigastric pain.
Skin: rash.

CHEM NAME	TRADE NAME	FORMULATION
naftidrofuryl oxalate	PRAXILENE	100mg
1–2 three times daily.		

SELECTIVE ALPHA BLOCKER

At this dosage and for this condition these are Category II drugs. See hypertension on pagec 110 for fuller details.

CHEM NAME	TRADE NAME	FORMULATION
prazosin	HYPOVASE	500mcg
Maintenance 2–4 twice daily.		
thymoxamine	OPILON	40mg
1 four times daily.		

VITAMIN E

Category II drug.
In general this is harmless if taken in physiological doses. However because it is fat soluble it tends to accumulate in the body. At very high doses it is toxic.
Effects:
Cardiovascular: thrombophlebitis.
Gastrointestinal: abdominal discomfort.
Blood: raised cholesterol levels.
Skin: rashes.

CHEM NAME	TRADE NAME	FORMULATION
Vitamin E	VITA-E-GELS	50, 75, 200 and 400 (all international units)
400–1600 i.u. daily.		

XANTHINE

Category II drug.
Precautions:
This drug must be used with caution in those with low blood pressure, severe ischaemic heart disease and renal disease.
Effects:
Gastrointestinal: nausea, indigestion.
Central nervous system: vertigo.
Skin: flushes.

CHEM NAME	TRADE NAME	FORMULATION
oxpentifylline	TRENTAL	400mg
1 two or three times daily.		

8   RESPIRATORY SYSTEM

NASAL CONDITIONS

Diseases treated by the drugs below are usually the allergic conditions affecting the nose such as allergic and perennial rhinitis.

ANTICHOLINERGIC

Category II.
   Also used in the treatment of asthma. See asthma on page 166 for full details.

CHEM NAME	TRADE NAME	FORMULATION
ipratropium	RINATEC	20mcg per dose (spray)

1–2 doses to each nostril up to four times daily.

SYMPATHOMIMETIC AGENTS

Category II.
Also used in cough remedies. See asthma on page 166 for full details.

CHEM NAME	TRADE NAME	FORMULATION
oxymetazoline	AFRAZINE	0.5mg per ml (spray and drops)

2–3 sprays or drops in each nostril twice daily.
Children: under 5 years, use paediatric drops, 5–12 years same as adult.

	VIBROCIL	0.25% with dimethindene, neomycin (drops, spray and gel)

3 sprays or 3–4 drops or a small quantity of gel in each nostril three or four times daily.
Children: under 6 years 1–2 drops in each nostril three or four times daily, 6–12 years, 3–4 drops in each nostril three or four times daily.
All ages, apply a small quantity of gel two or three times daily. With the addition of a sympathomimetic agent and an antihistamine. This drug can cause local irritation.

xylometazoline	OTRIVINE	0.1% (drops and spray)

Adults: 2–3 drops or 1–2 sprays in each nostril two or three times daily.

Children: use paediatric drops.

OTRIVINE PAED.   0.05% (drops)

Children over 3 months: 1–2 drops in each nostril once or twice daily.

MAST CELL STABILISER

Category II although if the patient is extremely allergic it may be more appropriate to consider it in Category III.

Also used in the treatment of asthma. See asthma on page 166 for full details.

CHEM NAME	TRADE NAME	FORMULATION
sodium cromoglycate	RYNACROM	2% (nasal spray)

Adults and children: 1 dose to each nostril four to six times daily. Therapy should be continuous.

RYNACROM NASAL 2%
DROPS

Adults and children: 2 drops in each nostril six times daily. Therapy should be continuous.

RYNACROM   2% with xylometazoline
COMPOUND   (spray)

Adults and children: 1 dose to each nostril four times daily.

With the addition of a sympathomimetic agent.

CORTICOSTEROID

Category III drugs.

Suppressive effects may lead to the development of more severe disease typically asthma and other respiratory complaints.

The use of any compound regularly to suppress a nasal discharge is potentially harmful.

For full details of corticosteroid treatment see page 258. Local application may also lead to adrenal suppression and so withdrawal must be slow.

General symptoms of corticosteroid use may be seen as with oral medication. Other symptoms of local use include nasal stinging, atrophic changes, throat irritation, atrophy of the nasal mucosa, Candidal and other fungal infections and nose bleeds.

CHEM NAME	TRADE NAME	FORMULATION
beclomethasone	BECONASE	50mcg per dose (aerosol)

2 applications in each nostril twice daily. Therapy should be continuous.
Children: under 6 years not recommended, 6–12 years adult dose.

betamethasone	BETNESOL	0.1% (drops)
	VISTA-METHASONE	0.1% (drops)
	BETNESOL-N	0.1% with 0.5% neomycin (drops)

With the addition of an antibiotic.

	VISTA-METHASONE N	0.1% with 0.5% neomycin (drops)

With the addition of an antibiotic.
Adults and children: 2–3 drops in each nostril two or three times daily.

budesonide	RHINOCORT	50mcg per dose (aerosol)

Maintenance 1 application in each nostril twice daily.
Children: not recommended for continuous long-term treatment.

dexamethasone	DEXA-RHINASPRAY	with tramazoline, neomycin (aerosol)

1 dose in each nostril up to maximum of 6 times in 24 hours.
With the addition of an antibiotic and a sympathomimetic.

flunisolide	SYNTARIS	25mcg per dose (spray)

Maximum of three times daily, reducing to minimum effective dose.
Therapy should be continuous.
Children: under 5 years, not recommended, 5–12 years, 1 spray in each nostril three times daily.

COMMENTS

The corticosteroids are clearly the most powerful of these drugs. The antihistamines and sympathomimetics have a local effect in drying secretions. They do not seem to have as many systemic side-effects as they do when taken orally.
Table of drugs listed in order of increasing strength:

CATEGORY II
- antihistamine
- sympathomimetic agent
CATEGORY II or III
- mast cell stabiliser
CATEGORY III

- corticosteroid

Any drug used to suppress a discharge, may, on its reduction, result in the appearance of the discharge usually worse than the original situation. In addition such suppression may well lead to the development of more severe disease. In this case the common result is the occurrence of respiratory disease such as asthma or bronchitis.

Withdrawal should be slow and treatment with alternative medicine used to help with the severe features which may result.

Allergic Disease

There are many types of allergic disease. Often the upper respiratory tract is affected as in allergic rhinitis (hay fever) but other cases include skin conditions, food reactions, drug reactions. Most treatment is aimed at reducing the worst effects so antihistamines are given to counteract the release of histamine — one of the main chemicals involved. Others may be used to try to prevent such release — mast cell stabilisers. Whatever approach is taken conventionally there is variable effect.

ANTIHISTAMINE

Category II drugs unless they are given to patients with severe manifestations of allergy in which case they are more appropriate in Category III (or even V in those with a risk of anaphylaxis). There are many different types of antihistamine on the market today. Some newer compounds are advertised as being free from the universal effect of drowsiness. However in my experience they may all cause tiredness and sedation. Adverse reactions are common and are seen in 50% of patients. Withdrawal of antihistamines may lead to the development of dyskinesia.

Contraindications:

Coma or central nervous system depression of any cause, those hypersensitive to phenothiazines, those taking MAOI or within two weeks of their administration.

Precautions:

This drug may thicken or dry lung secretions and so should be used with care in patients with asthma, bronchitis or bronchiectasis. Caution in severe coronary artery disease, narrow angle glaucoma, epilepsy, hepatic or renal insufficiency, prostate disease and hypertension.

Effects:

The elderly and very young are particularly sensitive.

General: drowsiness, tiredness, fever.

Cardiovascular: palpitations, hypotension, hypertension.

Central nervous system: dizziness, headaches, Parkinsonian-like symptoms of rigidity, weakness and tremor, tic-like movements of head and neck, muscle spasms, EEG changes, facial dyskinesia.

Psychological: restlessness, nightmares, disorientation, hallucinations, insomnia, irritability.

Gastrointestinal: dry mouth, nausea, vomiting, increased appetite, anorexia, epigastric pain, diarrhoea, constipation, jaundice.

Urogenital: urinary retention.

Allergy: anaphylaxis.

Blood disorders: haemolytic anaemia, agranulocytosis, thrombocytopenia, aplastic anaemia.

Skin: photosensitive reactions. Local use can lead to a contact dermatitis.

Special senses: blurred vision, nasal stuffiness.

CHEM NAME	TRADE NAME	FORMULATION
acrivastine	SEMPREX	8mg

1 three times daily.
Not for the elderly or children.

astemizole	HISMANAL	10mg, 5mg/5ml

1 tablet or 10ml daily.
Children: under 6 years not recommended, 6–12 years half adult dose.

azatadine	OPTIMINE	1mg, 0.5mg/5ml

1–2 tablets or 10–20ml twice daily.
Children: under 1 year not recommended, 1–6 years 2.5ml twice daily, 6–12 years 5–10ml twice daily.

	CONGESTEZE	1mg with 120mg pseudoephedrine

1 twice daily.
Children: not recommended.
With the addition of a sympathomimetic agent.

brompheniramine	DIMOTANE LA	12mg sustained-release

1–2 twice daily.
Children: under 6 years use elixir, 6–12 years 1 twice daily.

	DIMOTANE TABS.	4mg

DIMOTANE ELIXIR   2mg/5ml
1–2 tablet or 10–20ml three or four times daily.
Children: under 3 years 0.4–1mg/Kg daily, 3–6 years 5ml three or four times daily, 6–12 years half adult dose.

DIMOTANE PLUS   4mg/5ml with 30mg pseudoephedrine
10ml three times daily.
Children: under 6 years use paediatric elixir, 6–12 years 5ml three times daily.
With the addition of a sympathomimetic agent.

DIMOTANE PLUS   2mg/5ml with 15mg
PAEDIATRIC   pseudoephedrine
Children: under 2 years not recommended, 2–6 years 5ml three times daily, 6–12 years 10ml three times daily.
With the addition of a sympathomimetic agent.

DIMOTANE PLUS LA 12mg with 120mg pseudoephedrine sustained-release
1 twice daily.
Children: not recommended.

cetirizine   ZIRTEK   10mg
1 daily.
Children: not recommended.

chlor-   PIRITON   4mg, 2mg/5ml
  pheniramine
4mg three or four times daily.
Children: up to 1 year 2.5ml twice daily, 1–5 years 2.5–5ml three times daily, over 5 years 5–10ml or ½–1 tab. three or four times daily.

PIRITON   12mg sustained-release
SPANDETS
1 two to three times daily.

HAYMINE   10mg with 15mg ephedrine
1–2 daily.
Children: not recommended. With the addition of a sympathomimetic agent.

clemastine   TAVEGIL   1mg, 0.5mg/5ml
1 tablet or 10ml twice daily.
Children: ½–1 tab. or 5–10ml twice daily.

cyproheptadine   PERIACTIN   4mg, 2mg/5ml
4mg three or four times daily.
Children: under 2 years not recommended, 2–6 years 2mg, 7–14 years 4mg. Both three times daily.
This drug may cause a toxic psychosis. It goes with stopping the drug.

dimethindene	FENOSTIL RETARD	2.5mg sustained-release

1 twice daily.
Children: not recommended.

diphenyl-
  pyraline
	HISTRYL
	  SPANSULE
		5mg sustained-release

	LERGOBAN	5mg sustained-release

1–2 twice daily.

	HISTRYL PAED.	2.5mg sustained-release

Children: under 7 years not recommended, over 7 years 1 twice daily.

loratadine	CLARITYN	10mg

1 daily.
Not for the elderly or children.

mebhydrolin	FABAHISTIN	50mg, 50mg/5ml

50–100mg three times daily.
Children: 5–20ml daily.
This drug may cause a granulocytopenia.

mequitazine	PRIMALAN	5mg

1 twice daily.
Children: not recommended.
This drug is related to the phenothiazines and may cause similar
effects as that group (see page 93).

oxatomide	TINSET	30mg

1–2 twice daily.
Children: under 5 years not recommended, over 5 years half adult
dose.

phenindamine	THEPHORIN	25mg

1–2 one to three times daily.
Children: not recommended.

pheniramine	DANERAL SA	75mg sustained–release

1–2 at night.
Children: not recommended.

promethazine	PHENERGAN	10mg, 25mg, 5mg/5ml

10–20mg two or three times daily.
Children: under 1 year not recommended, 1–5 years 5–15mg, over 5
years 10–25mg.

terfenadine	TRILUDAN	60mg, 30mg/5ml
	TRILUDAN FORTE	120mg

60mg twice daily or 120mg once daily.
Children: under 6 years not recommended, 6–12 years 30mg twice
daily.

trimeprazine	VALLERGAN	10mg, 7.5mg/5ml
	VALLERGAN FORTE SYRUP	30mg/5ml

10mg three or four times daily.

Children: under 2 years not recommended, over 2 years 2.5–5mg three or four times daily.

| triprolidine | ACTIDIL | 2.5mg, 2mg/5ml |

1–2 tablets or 5–10ml three times daily.
Children: under 1 year 2.5ml, 1–6 years 5ml, 6–12 years 7.5ml. All three times daily.

| | PRO-ACTIDIL | 10mg sustained-release |

1 daily.
Children: not recommended.

| | SUDAFED PLUS | 2.5mg with 60mg pseudoephedrine |
| | SUDAFED PLUS SYRUP | 1.25mg/5ml with 30mg pseudoephedrine |

1 tablet or 10ml three times daily.
Children: under 2 years not recommended, 2–5 years 2.5ml three times daily, 6–12 years 5ml three times daily.
With the addition of a sympathomimetic agent.

COMMENTS

These drugs are of variable effectiveness in removing the symptoms of allergic conditions. Despite claims to the contrary they may all produce tiredness. Treating patients who take these drugs can be very difficult because it necessitates the reappearance of the allergic state.
Table of drugs in order of increasing strength:

CATEGORY II
- antihistamine
- antihistamine plus sympathomimetic agent
CATEGORY III or V
- antihistmines used to treat severe and serious manifestations of allergic disease

The expected withdrawal symptoms are anxiety, restlessness, insomnia as the sedating effects of the drug are removed. Allergic symptoms of the presenting condition will appear and these should be treated as necessary. If the drug is taken for a condition such as hay fever which only appears during the season then take care that the drug is not stopped too quickly before the pollen season. The patient may feel all is well only for problems to occur when the hay fever season fully develops.

Most people who have regular attacks of hay fever have an

underlying condition which needs to be treated constitutionally. Only then will the recurrent attacks of allergic manifestations subside.

Antihistamines are also used in children with sleep or behavioural disorders where their sedating effects are used.

MAST CELL STABILISER

This is usually Category II unless the patient is very allergic in which case it would be more appropriate to place in Category III.

Also used in the treatment of asthma. See asthma for details. These mask the symptoms of allergy to a variable degree. Many patients view them with disdain because they may be particularly ineffective.

Reduction may be necessary to 'see' the clinical picture. When this appears a diagnosis can be made and treatment begun.

CHEM NAME	TRADE NAME	FORMULATION
ketotifen	ZADITEN	1mg, 1mg/5ml

1–2mg twice daily.
Children: under 2 years not recommended, over 2 years 1 mg twice daily.

sodium cromoglycate	NALCROM	100mg

2 four times daily.
Children: under 2 years not recommended, over 2 years half adult dose.

Cough Remedies

All the cough remedies listed below are either in Category I (symptomatic use) or Category II (regular use).

These are used for a variety of coughs. In general, coughs which are dry are suppressed by means of morphine derivatives such as codeine. Coughs which produce mucus are encouraged by means of menthol, eucalyptus and other expectorants.

There may also be a variety of other chemicals such as antihistamines, sympathomimetics, caffeine. There is no real evidence even conventionally that these mixtures of drugs have any advantage over a simple linctus. They may of course do a lot of harm particularly if taken in large amounts, for prolonged periods or in sensitive individuals.

Despite the above you will often find that remedies may contain expectorants or demulcents to help cough up mucus together with opiates which are designed to suppress cough. There is a singular lack of logic here.

There are probably more remedies available over-the-counter than are listed here. It can be instructive to visit your local pharmacy and see how many are available.

EXPECTORANT

This aids coughing. It is unlikely to lead to problems. High doses may cause nausea and/or vomiting.

CHEM NAME	TRADE NAME	FORMULATION
ammonium chloride	AMMONIUM CHLORIDE MIXTURE	

10–20ml three or four times daily.
Children: not recommended.

	GUANOR	with sodium citrate, 14mg diphenhydramine, menthol

5–10ml every two or three hours.
Children: under 1 year not recommended, 1–5 years 2.5ml, 6–12 years 5ml. Both three or four hourly.
With the addition of an antihistamine and a demulcent.

acetylcysteine	FABROL	200mg granules (sachets)

1 sachet three times daily.
Children: under 2 years 1 daily, 2–6 years 1 twice daily, over 6 years adult dose.
This drug may lead to nausea, heartburn, vomiting, nettle rash, headache, tinnitus and wheezing (particularly in asthmatic patients).

MUCOLYTIC

This is designed to thin sputum.

CHEM NAME	TRADE NAME	FORMULATION
carbocisteine	MUCODYNE	250mg/5ml

15ml three times daily reducing to 10ml three times daily.
Children: use Paed.

	MUCODYNE CAPS.	375mg

One four times daily.

	MUCODYNE PAED.	125mg/5ml

Children: under 2 years not recommended, 2–5 years 2.5–5ml four timesdaily, 5–12 years 10ml three times daily.

methylcysteine	VISCLAIR	100mg

2 three or four times daily for 6 weeks then 2 twice daily.
Children: under 5 years not recommended, over 5 years 1 three times daily.

ANTIHISTAMINE

See allergic disease on page 157 for details.

CHEM NAME	TRADE NAME	FORMULATION
brompheniramine	DIMOTANE EXPECTORANT	2mg with guaiphenesin, 30mg pseudoephedrine/5ml

5–10ml three times daily.
Children: under 2 years not recommended, 2–6 years 2.5ml, 6–12 years 5ml. Both three times daily.
With the addition of an expectorant and a sympathomimetic agent.

	DIMOTANE CO	2mg with 10mg codeine phosphate, 30mg pseudoephedrine/5ml

10ml three times daily.
Children: under 6 years use the Paediatric formula, over 6 years 7.5ml three times daily.
With the addition of an opiate and a sympathomimetic agent.

	DIMOTANE CO PAED.	2mg with 3mg codeine phosphate 15mg pseudoephedrine/5ml

Children: under 2 years not recommended, 2–3 years 5ml, 3–6 years 10ml, 6–12 years 15ml. All three times daily.
With the addition of an opiate and a sympathomimetic agent.

| | DIMOTAPP LA | 12mg with 15mg phenylephrine, 15mg phenylpropanolamine sustained-release |

1–2 night and morning.
Children: use elixir.
With the addition of sympathomimetic agents.

| | DIMOTAPP ELIXIR | 4mg with 5mg phenylpropanolamine, 5mg phenylephrine/5ml |

5–10ml three times daily.
Children: under 2 years not recommended, 2–6 years 2.5–5ml, 6–12 years 5ml. Both three times daily.
With the addition of sympathomimetic agents.

| | DIMOTAPP ELIXIR PAED. | 1mg with 2.5mg phenyl-propanolamine 2.5mg phenylephrine/5ml |

Children: under 2 years not recommended, 2–6 years 2.5–10ml, 6–12 years 10ml. Both three times daily.
With the addition of sympathomimetic agents.

| carbinoxamine | DAVENOL | 2mg with 7mg ephedrine, 4mg pholcodine/5ml |

5–10ml three or four times daily.
Children: up to 5ml three or four times daily.
With the addition of a sympathomimetic agent and an opiate.

| diphenhydramine | BENYLIN Chesty Cough | 14mg/5ml with ammonium chloride, sodium citrate, menthol |

5–10ml two to three hourly.
Children: under 1 year not recommended, 1–5 years 2.5ml, 6–12 years 5ml. Both three or four hourly.
With the addition of an expectorant and demulcents.

| | BENYLIN Children's Cough | 7mg/5ml with sodium citrate, menthol |

Children: under 1 year not recommended, 1–5 years 5ml, over 6 years 10ml. Both every three hours.
With demulcents.

| | BENYLIN DECONGESTANT | 14mg/5ml with menthol, 10mg pseudoephedrine, sodium citrate |

10ml four times daily.
Children: under 1 year not recommended, 1–5 years quarter adult dose, 6–12 years half adult dose.
With the addition of a sympathomimetic agent and a demulcent.

| | BENYLIN with CODEINE | 14mg/5ml with 5.7mg codeine phosphate, |

sodium citrate, menthol

10ml three or four hourly.
Children: under 1 year not recommended, 1–5 years quarter adult dose, 6–12 years half adult dose.
With the addition of an opiate and demulcents.

HISTALIX   14mg/5ml with
             ammonium chloride,
             sodium citrate, menthol

5–10ml three hourly.
Children: half adult dose.
With the addition of an expectorant and demulcents.

LOTUSSIN   5mg/5ml with 6.25mg
             dextromethorphan

10ml three times daily.
Children: under 1 year not recommended, 1–5 years 2.5–5ml, 6–12 years 5–10ml. Both three times daily.
With the addition of an opiate.

promethazine   PHENSEDYL   3.6mg/5ml with 9mg
                               codeine phosphate

5–10ml twice or three times daily.
Children: under 2 years not recommended, 2–5 years 2.5ml, over 5 years 2.5–5ml. Both twice or three times daily.
With the addition of an opiate.

triprolidine   ACTIFED CO.   1.25mg/5ml with 30mg
                                 pseudoephedrine, 10mg
                                 dextromethorphan

With the addition of a sympathomimetic agent and an opiate.

ACTIFED   1.25mg with 30mg
EXPECTORANT   pseudoephedrine,
                 guaiphenesin

10ml three times daily.
Children: under 2 not recommended, 2–5 years 2.5ml, 6–12 years 5ml. Both three times daily.
With the addition a sympathomimetic agent and an expectorant.

ACTIFED TABS.   2.5mg with 60mg
                  pseudoephedrine

ACTIFED SYRUP   10ml = 1 tablet

1 tab. or 10ml three times daily.
Children: under 2 years not recommended, 2–5 years 2.5ml, 6–12 years 5ml. Both three times daily.
With the addition of a sympathomimetic agent.

OPIATE

These are derived from the opium poppy and heroin is the most powerful example. They are commonly used analgesics and are described in more detail in page 213.

They are used to sedate the cough. It will also sedate the patient and lead to drowsiness as well as the possibility of addiction.

CHEM NAME	TRADE NAME	FORMULATION
codeine phosphate	GALCODINE	15mg/5ml

5ml four times daily.
Children: under 1 year not recommended, 1–5 years 2.5–5ml, 6–12 years 5ml. Both three or four times daily.

	GALCODINE PAED.	3mg/5ml

Children: under 1 year not recommended, 1–5 years 5ml three or four times daily, 6–12 years use ordinary linctus.

	TERCODA	8mg/5ml with terpin, cineole, menthol, peppermint oil, pine oil/5ml

5–10ml three times daily.
Children: not recommended.
With the addition of expectorants and demulcents.

	TERPOIN	15mg/5ml with cineole, menthol

5ml three hourly.
Children: not recommended.
With the addition of demulcents.

	UNIFLU AND GREGOVITE C	10 mg with 500mg para-cetamol, 30mg caffeine, 15mg diphenhydramine, 10mg phenylephrine (GREGOVITE C = Vit.C)

1 of each every four hours.
Maximum 6 in 24 hours.
Children: not recommended.
With the addition of a paracetamol analgesic, xanthine, antihistamine, sympathomimetic agents and Vitamin C.

NOTE: XANTHINES are stimulants used in the form of theophylline for asthma. Here caffeine is the example.
It is a mild stimulant which is often added to cough remedies,
analgesics and the like. It probably does not aid their action and
it is difficult to see the rationale behind its use. It may also be
used on its own to ward off tiredness.
Withdrawal of caffeine leads to restlessness, headache and
irritability.
Effects:
Cardiovascular: palpitations, raised blood pressure, may
increase the risk of myocardial infarction in women if they
drink 6 or more cups of coffee per day.
Gastrointestinal: increases gastric irritation of aspirin, nausea,
vomiting, exacerbates duodenal ulcer because leads to increase
in gastric acid secretion (decaffeinated coffee has the same
effect here as 'regular' coffee), carcinoma of pancreas.
Psychological: insomnia, anxiety, feelings of tension, irritability, psychosis.
Endocrine: hyperglycaemia.
Urogenital: excessive urination. It may add to the renal damage
caused by analgesics.
Skin: urticaria.

CHEM NAME	TRADE NAME	FORMULATION
dihydrocodeine	DF118	10mg/5ml

5ml four to six hourly after meals.
Children: under 4 years not recommended, 4–12 years 0.2mg/Kg body
weight every four to six hours.

	PARAMOL	10mg with 500mg paracetamol

1 four hourly.
Children: not recommended.
With the addition of a paracetamol analgesic.

pholcodine	COPHOLCO	5.63mg with menthol, cineole, terpin/5ml

10ml four to five times daily.
Children: under 5 years not recommended, over 5 years 2.5–5ml four
to five times daily.
With the addition of expectorants.

	COPHOLCOIDS	4mg with menthol, cineole, terpin

1–2 three or four times daily.

Children: under 5 years not recommended, over 5 years 1 three times daily.

With the addition of expectorants.

| EXPULIN | 5mg/5ml with 15mg pseudoephedrine, 2mg chlorpheniramine, menthol |

10ml four times daily.

Children: under 2 years use Paed. linctus, 2–6 years 2.5–5ml, 6–12 years 5–10ml. Both four times daily.

With the addition of a sympathomimetic agent, antihistamine and a demulcent.

| EXPULIN PAED. | 2mg/5ml with 1mg chlorpheniramine, menthol |

Children: under 1 year not recommended, 1–3 years 5ml, 3–10 years 10ml. Both twice or three times daily.

With the addition of antihistamine and a demulcent.

| GALENPHOL | 5mg/5ml |

5–10ml three or four times daily.

Children: under 1 year not recommended, 1–5 years 2.5–5ml, 6–12 years 5ml. Both three or four times daily.

| GALENPHOL LINCTUS STRONG | 10mg/5ml |

5ml three or four times daily.

Children: not recommended.

| GALENPHOL LINCTUS PAED. | 2mg/5ml |

Children under 3 months not recommended, 3–12 months 2.5ml, 1–5 years 5–10ml, 6–12 years 10ml. All three times daily.

| PAVACOL-D | 5mg/5ml with aromatic and volatile oiis |

5–10ml as necessary.

Children: under 1 year not recommended, 1–2 years 2.5ml three or four times daily, 3–5 years 5ml three times daily, 6–12 years 5ml four to five times daily.

With the addition of demulcents.

| PHOLCOMED-D | 5mg/5ml with 1.25mg papaverine |

10–15ml three or four times daily.

Children: under 1 year not recommended, 1–2 years 2.5ml, over 2 years 5ml. Both three times daily.

With the addition of a bronchorelaxant.

| PHOLCOMED-D FORTE | 19mg/5ml with 5mg papaverine |

5ml three times daily after meals.

Children: not recommended.
With the addition of a bronchorelaxant.

	PHOLCOMED PASTILLES	4mg/5ml with 1mg papaverine

Up to 2 every hour. Maximum 15 daily.
Children: 1 hourly. Maximum 7 daily.
With the addition of a bronchorelaxant.

SYMPATHOMIMETIC AGENT

These are used in many situations including asthma. They are a common constituent of cough and cold remedies because they help to dry secretions. There are many formulations sold over-the-counter and include remedies for hay fever and eye drops. See asthma on page 166 for full details.

CHEM NAME	TRADE NAME	FORMULATION
ephedrine	EXPURHIN	4mg/5ml with 1mg chlorpheniramine

Children: under 3 months not recommended, 3–12 months 2.5–5ml twice daily, 1–5 years 5–10ml three times daily, 6–12 years 10–15ml three times daily.
With the addition of an antihistamine.

phenyl-propanolamine	ESKORNADE SPANSULE	50mg with 5mg diphenyl-pyraline sustained-release

1 twelve hourly.
With the addition of an antihistamine.

	ESKORNADE SYRUP	12.5mg/5ml with 1.5mg diphenylpyraline

10ml up to four times daily.
Children: under 2 years not recommended, 2–5 years one quarter adult dose, over 6 years half adult dose.
With the addition of an antihistamine.

pseudoephedrine	GALPSEUD	60mg

1 three times daily.

	GALPSEUD LINCTUS	30mg/5ml

10ml three times daily.
Children: under 2 years not recommended, 2–6 years 2.5ml three or four times daily, 6–12 years 5ml three or four times daily.

	SUDAFED	60mg, 30mg/5ml

1 tab. or 10ml three times daily.

Children: under 2 years not recommended, 2–5 years 2.5ml, 6–12 years 5ml. Both three times daily.

	SUDAFED SA	120mg sustained-release

1 twice daily.

	SUDAFED-CO	60mg with 500mg paracetamol

1 three times daily.

Children: under 6 years not recommended, over 6 years half adult dose.

With the addition of a paracetamol analgesic.

	SUDAFED EXPECTORANT	30mg with guaiphenesin

10ml three times daily.

Children: under 2 years not recommended, 2–5 years 2.5ml, 6–12 years 5ml. Both three times daily.

With the addition of an expectorant.

This drug causes rashes and may lead to raised blood pressure especially in children.

ANTITUSSIVE

This aims to reduce coughing.

CHEM NAME	TRADE NAME	FORMULATION
isoaminile	ISOAMINILE LINCTUS	40mg/5ml

5ml three to five times daily.

Children: 2.5–5ml three to five times daily.

SELECTIVE BETA-AGONIST

These are commonly used in the treatment of asthma. See asthma on page 166 for full details.

CHEM NAME	TRADE NAME	FORMULATION
terbutaline	BRICANYL Expectorant	1.5mg with guaiphenesin

10–15ml eight hourly.

Not for children.

With the addition of an expectorant.

COMMENTS

There are many substances prescribed and available over-the-counter for coughs and colds. Most contain mixtures of compounds reputed to relieve dry throat, runny nose, dry cough, cough with sputum, and so on.

However, there are some chemicals, i.e. antihistamine, sympathomimetics, opiates which have more general actions and may lead to general symptoms.

Table of drugs in order of increasing strength:

CATEGORY I (symptomatic use) or CATEGORY II (regular use)
- mucolytic, demulcent and the like
- antihistamine
- sympathomimetics
- selective beta agonist
- opiates

When dealing with these agents there should be little problem when they are taken symptomatically. People can be educated to take remedies which are less hazardous — herbal or homoeopathic formulations and use will stop when the condition improves.

When there is regular medication for a more chronic condition such as chronic bronchitis then there will more of a problem for the practitioner.

The expected reaction will depend on the particular drug taken. Check the withdrawal effects under the details for each drug.

Asthma

Asthma is very common. It is seen in both children and adults and may have an allergic component particularly in younger patients with so-called 'atopy'. The basis of treatment is with drugs although patients may also be given advice about exercise and breathing.

There are increasing moves to treat asthma 'aggressively'. That is to start treatment earlier, for milder cases and to use corticosteroid inhalers at the beginning of treatment rather than wait to see the effect of bronchodilators.

Other diseases with wheezing such as chronic bronchitis and emphysema may also be treated with these drugs but with limited results. The feature of asthma is that the wheezing is reversible rather than the more permanent type seen in more chronic lung disease.

SYMPATHOMIMETICS

Category II drugs.

Adrenaline is the main example of this group of drugs but this is no longer used for asthma because of its severe effects. Its common prescription in the 1950s was related to an increasing death rate.

They have a stimulant effect, produce an adrenaline-like response and so have similar effects to amphetamines ('speed'). It is this effect which serves to 'stimulate' the lungs and so relieve the symptom of wheezing.

They tend to worsen conditions such as epilepsy, hypertension and anxiety.

Contraindications:

Severe hypertension, severe coronary artery disease and those taking MAOI or within two weeks of their administration.

Effects:

Systemic effects are seen even if taken as nasal sprays or drops. Thyrotoxic patients are especially susceptible to the effects.

General: tremor.

Cardiovascular: increased heart rate, palpitations which may precipitate angina.

Psychological: insomnia, anxiety, sedation in children, sleep disturbances, psychosis, hallucinations.

Urogenital: urinary retention, dysuria.

Skin: rashes.

CHEM NAME	TRADE NAME	FORMULATION
ephedrine	CAM	4mg/5ml with butethamate

20ml three or four times daily.
Children: under 3 months not recommended, 3 months–2 years 2.5ml, 2–4 years, 5ml, over 4 years, 10ml. All three times daily.
With the addition of an anticholinergic agent.

	FRANOL	11mg with 120mg theophylline
	FRANOL PLUS	15mg with 120mg theophylline

1 three times daily and at bedtime if required.
Not for children.

With the addition of a xanthine.

XANTHINES

Category II drugs.
Drugs such as aminophylline, theophylline, choline theophyllinate and diprophylline are commonly given for wheezing attacks or on a regular basis to prevent attacks.
They are very powerful drugs and it is important that their use is closely monitored. This should be by means of serum levels, clinical condition and questioning about adverse effects. These three are hardly ever done in my experience.
Contraindications:
They should not be given with ephedrine in children. This will be of importance both for prescribed drugs which contain ephedrine as well as over-the-counter remedies for coughs and colds, many of which contain ephedrine.
Precautions:
The dosage in the elderly should be reduced by 25% (50% if there are signs of cardiac failure). Liver disease will increase the effects of the drugs because 90% of the drug is metabolised by that organ.
Effects:
General: tremor.
Cardiovascular: palpitations, rapid heart rate, hypotension, arrhythmias (may be fatal especially if pre-existing heart disease).
Gastrointestinal: nausea, vomiting, indigestion.
Central nervous system: headache, dizziness, convulsions.
Psychological: anxiety, agitation, insomnia, confusion, psychosis.
Blood: thrombocytopenia.
Skin: rash, pruritus.
Special senses: visual disturbances.

CHEM NAME	TRADE NAME	FORMULATION
aminophylline	PECRAM	225mg sustained-release
1 twice daily.		
	PHYLLOCONTIN CONTINUS	225mg sustained-release
Maintenance 2 twice daily.		

	PHYLLOCONTIN FORTE	350mg sustained-release

1 or 2 twice daily.

	PHYLLOCONTIN PAEDIATRIC	100mg sustained-release

Children: not for under 1 year. Over 1 year, 12mg/Kg twice daily.

THEO-DROX	195mg with aluminium hydroxide

1 four times daily.
With the addition of an antacid.
This drug may worsen wheezing.

choline	CHOLEDYL	100mg, 200mg, 62.5mg/5ml

theophyllinate
100–400mg four times daily.
Children: Under 3 years not recommended, 3–6 years 5–10ml three times daily, 6–12 years: 100mg three or four times daily.

SABIDAL SR	270mg sustained-release

2 at night and 1 in the morning. Not to be given to children.

theophylline	BIOPHYLLINE	350mg, 500mg, 125mg/ml

Over 70Kg 500mg, under 70Kg 350mg. Both twice daily.
5–10ml three to four times daily.
Children: Under 2 years not recommended, 2–6 years 2.5ml, 7–12 years 2.5–5ml. Both three to four times daily.

LASMA	300mg

1 twice daily. Increase by half tablets if required.
Children: not recommended.

NUELIN SA	175mg sustained-release

1–2 twice daily.
Children: Under 6 years not recommended, over 6 years 1 twice daily.

NUELIN SA-250	250mg sustained-release

1–2 twice daily.
Children: under 6 years not recommended, over 6 years half adult dose.

NUELIN	125mg

1–2 three or four times daily.
Children: under 7 years not recommended, 7–12 years half adult dose.

NUELIN LIQUID	60mg/5ml

10–20ml three or four times daily.
Children: Under 2 years not recommended, 2–6 years 5–7.5ml, 7–12 years 7.5–10ml. All three or four times daily.

PRO-VENT	300mg sustained-release

1 twice daily. Increase by 1 daily if necessary.
Not for children.

| | SLO-PHYLLIN | 60mg, 125mg, 250mg all sustained-release |

250–500mg twice daily.
Children: under 2 years not recommended, 2–6 years 60–120mg, 6–12 years 125–250mg. Both twice daily.

| | THEO-DUR | 200mg, 300mg both sustained-release |

200mg or 300mg twice daily to begin.
Children: under 35Kg 100mg, over 35Kg 200mg. Both twice daily.

| | UNIPHYLLIN CONTINUS | 300mg, 400mg both sustained-release |

Less than 70Kg 300mg twice daily. Over 70Kg 400mg twice daily.
Children: use Paediatric formulation.

| | UNIPHYLLIN PAEDIATRIC CONTINUS | 200mg sustained-release |

Children: under 5 year not recommended, 5–9 years (10–28Kg) 9mg/Kg twice daily, over 9 years (over 28Kg) as adult.

BETA AGONISTS

Category II drugs.
These are of differing types, some are specific for certain groups of receptors, others less so. They are used for their bronchodilating effect.
Precautions:
Thyrotoxicosis, myocardial insufficiency, angina, cardiac arrhythmias, hypertension, diabetes mellitus. As 50% is excreted via the kidney caution must be taken in renal disease. Concurrent use of MAOI or tricyclic antidepressants or sympathomimetic agents. These drugs may lead to lead to the prolongation of pregnancy and inhibition of labour.
Effects:
Cardiovascular: palpitations, rapid pulse rate.
Central nervous system: tremor.

CHEM NAME	TRADE NAME	FORMULATION
fenoterol	BEROTEC	inhaler (0.2mg/dose)

1 or 2 puffs three times daily, maximum 2 puffs four hourly.
Children: 1 puff three times daily, maximum 1 puff four hourly.

| | DUOVENT | inhaler (0.1mg/dose) with |

ipratropium

1–2 puffs three or four times daily.
Children: Under 6 years, not recommended, over 6 years, 1 puff three
times daily.
With the addition of an anticholinergic agent.

| isoetharine | NUMOTAC | 10mg sustained-release |

1–2 three or four times daily.
Children: not recommended.

| | BRONCHILATOR | inhaler (350mcg/dose) |
| | | with phenylephrine |

1 or 2 puffs repeated after 30 minutes if necessary. Maximum 16 puffs
in 24 hours.
Children: not recommended.
With the addition of a sympathomimetic agent.

isoprenaline	ISO-AUTOHALER	inhaler (0.08mg/dose)
	MEDIHALER-ISO	inhaler (0.08mg/dose)
	DUO-AUTOHALER	inhaler (0.16mg/dose)
		with phenylephrine

With the addition of a sympathomimetic agent

| | MEDI-HALER DUO | inhaler (0.16mg with |
| | | phenylephrine) |

1–2 puffs repeated after 30 minutes if necessary. Maximum 24 puffs in
24 hours. Same for adults and children.
With the addition of a sympathomimetic agent.

| orciprenaline | ALUPENT | 20mg, 10mg/5ml, inhaler |
| | | (0.75mg/dose) |

1 tablet or 10ml four times daily.
Inhaler: 1–2 puffs repeated every 30 minutes if necessary. Maximum
12 puffs in 24 hours.
Children: Up to 1 year, 2.5–5ml three times daily, 1–3 years, 2.5–5ml
four times daily, 3–12 years, 5ml four times daily to 10ml three times
daily.
Inhaler: under 6 years 1 puff, 6–12 years 1–2 puffs. Both not to be
repeated within 30 minutes. Maximum 4 puffs in 24 hours.

| pirbuterol | EXIREL | 10mg, 15mg, inhaler |
| | | (0.2mg/dose) |

Tablets: 10–15mg three or four times daily, maximum 60mg daily.
Not for children.
Inhaler: 2 puffs three or four times daily. Maximum 12 puffs daily.
Not for children.

| reproterol | BRONCHODIL | inhaler (0.5mg/dose), |
| | | 20mg |

1 or 2 puffs three to six hourly, prophylaxis, 1 puff three times daily.
20mg three times daily reducing to 10mg three times daily if
side-effects occur.
Children: Under 6 years, not recommended, 6–12 years, 1 puff three

to six hourly, prophylaxis, 1 puff three times daily. 10mg three times daily.

rimiterol	PULMADIL	inhaler (0.2mg/dose)
	PULMADIL AUTO	inhaler (0.2mg/dose)

1–3 doses repeated after 30 minutes if necessary. Maximum 24 doses in 24 hours. Same for adults and children.

salbutamol	AEROLIN	inhaler (100mcg/dose)
	AUTOHALER	

Inhaler: acute attack, 1–2 puffs. Prophylaxis, 2 puffs three or four times daily.
Children: half the adult dose.

	ASMAVEN	2mg, 4mg

Tablets: 2–4mg three or four times daily.
Elderly: initially 2mg three or four times daily.
Children: Tablets not recommended under 2 years, 2–6 years 1–2mg, 6–12 years, 2mg. Both orally three or four times daily.

	SALBULIN	4mg, inhaler
		(100mcg/dose)

Inhaler: acute attack, 1–2 puffs. Prophylaxis, 2 puffs three or four times daily.
Children: half adult dose.
Tablets: 2–4mg three or four times daily.
Children: Not for children.

	SALBUVENT	2mg, 4mg, 2mg/5ml,
		inhaler (100mcg/dose)

Inhaler: acute attack, 1–2 puffs. Prophylaxis, 2 puffs three or four times daily.
Children: half adult dose.
Tablets: 2–4mg three or four times daily.
Children: not recommended under 2 years, 2–6 years 1–2mg, 6–12 years, 2mg. Both three or four times daily.

	VENTODISKS	inhaler (200mcg or
		400mcg/dose)

Acute attack, 200 or 400mcg as a single dose. Prophylaxis, 400mcg three or four times daily.
Children: Acute, 200mcg, prophylaxis, half adult dose.

	VENTOLIN	2mg, 4mg, 2mg/5ml,
		inhaler (100mcg/dose)

Inhaler: acute attack, 1–2 puffs. Prophylaxis, 2 puffs three or four times daily.
Children: half adult dose.
Tablets: 2–4mg three or four times daily.
Children: not recommended under 2 years, 2–6 years 1–2mg, 6–12 years 2mg. Both three or four times daily.

	VENTOLIN CR	4mg, 8mg both

sustained-release

8mg twice daily.
Children: under 3 years not recommended, 3–12 years 4mg twice daily.

| | VENTOLIN ROTACAPS | inhaled as 200mcg and 400mcg/dose |

Acute attack, 200 or 400mcg as a single dose. Prophylaxis, 400mcg three or four times daily. Prophylaxis, 400mcg three or four times daily.
Children: Acute, 200mcg, prophylaxis, half adult dose.

| | VOLMAX | 4mg, 8mg both sustained-release |

8mg twice daily.
Children: under 3 years not recommended, 3–12 years 4mg twice daily.
This drug may cause hot feelings in the extremities, raised blood sugar, sweating and nausea. In those who take this drug excessively it may cause a decrease in oxygen levels.

| terbutaline | BRICANYL | 5mg, 1.5mg/5ml, inhaler (0.25mg/dose) 'turbohaler' 0.5mg/dose |
| | MONOVENT | 5mg, 1.5mg/5ml |

Tablets: 1 twice or three times daily.
Children: 7–15 years half adult dose.
Syrup: 10–15ml.
Children: Under 3 years 2.5ml, 3–7 years 2.5–5ml, 7–15 years 5–10ml. All three times daily.
Inhaler: 1–2 puffs as required. Maximum 8 puffs in 24 hours. Same dose for adults and children.
'Turbohaler': 1 inhalation as required. Maximum 4 in 24 hours. Same dose for adults and children.

| | BRICANYL SA | 7.5mg |
| | MONOVENT SA | 7.5mg |

1 twice daily.
Drowsiness is especially seen with this drug (in 25% of patients).

ANTICHOLINERGIC DRUGS

Category II drugs.
These are also used for many conditions including diarrhoea. In asthma they are bronchodilators.
As a group they block the action of acetylcholine (a parasympathetic nervous system neurotransmitter) so the the effect will basically be an adrenaline effect (a sympathetic nervous system neurotransmitter).

Contraindications:
Hypersensitivity to atropine.
Precautions:
Glaucoma or prostatic hypertrophy, fever, hot weather.
Effects:
General: drowsiness, drying of secretions, fever.
Cardiovascular: increased heart rate.
Gastrointestinal: dry mouth, thirst, vomiting, constipation.
Central nervous system: giddiness, slurred speech, convulsions.
Psychological: hallucinations, disorientation, confusion, memory impairment, restlessness, agitation, hyperactivity, apprehension, fear, paranoia.
Urogenital: urinary retention.
Skin: flushing, rash.

CHEM NAME	TRADE NAME	FORMULATION
ipratropium	ATROVENT	inhaler (0.02mg/dose)

1 or 2 puffs three or four times daily.
Children: Under 6 years, 1 puff, 6–12 years, 1 or 2 puffs. Both three times daily.

	ATROVENT FORTE	inhaler (0.04mg/dose)

1 or 2 puffs three or four times daily.
Children: Under 6 years, use standard inhaler, 6–12 years, usually 1 puff three times daily.

CORTICOSTEROIDS

Category III drugs.

Those listed here as inhalers are not associated with any great problems conventionally. However, they will be suppressive in the same way as oral forms and they are certainly absorbed into the systemic circulation leading to general effects. The conventional belief that they only affect the lung is nonsense. The effect of inhaled forms will be less than that of oral presentations.

They are given regularly to reduce inflammation in the lung, to help with problems caused by mucus and to relieve wheezing. These particular chemicals are also used for skin conditions and hay fever in different formulations.
Contraindications:
Hypersensitivity and allergy.

Precautions:
They must be taken regularly as they act as a prophylactic.
Caution in quiescent and active tuberculosis.
Effects:
Local problems of thrush of the throat or mouth. This occurs in
10% of patients.

CHEM NAME	TRADE NAME	FORMULATION
beclomethasone	BECLOFORTE	inhaler (250mcg/dose)

2 puffs three or four times daily if necessary.
Not for children.

	BECODISKS	inhaler (100, 200 or 400mcg/dose)

Usually 400mcg twice daily or 200mcg three or four times daily.
Maximum 1000mcg daily.
Children: 100mcg two to four times daily.

	BECOTIDE INHALER	inhaler (50 or 100mcg/ dose)

400mcg daily. Severe cases, initially 600–800mcg daily, reducing
according to response.
Children: 50–100mcg two to four times daily.

	BECOTIDE ROTACAPS	inhaled as 100, 200, 400mcg/dose

200mcg three or four times daily or 300–400mcg twice daily.
Children: 100mcg two to four times daily.

	BECOTIDE SUSPENSION	50mcg/ml

Children: Up to 1 year, 1ml, over 1 year, 2ml Both nebulised two to four
times daily.

	VENTIDE	inhaler (50mcg/dose) with 100mcg salbutamol

2 puffs three or four times daily.
Children: 1 or 2 puffs two to four times daily.
With the addition of a bronchodilator.

		rotacaps (200mcg/dose) with 400mcg salbutamol

1 three or four times daily.
With the addition of a bronchodilator.

		paediatric rotacaps (100mcg/dose) with 200mcg salbutamol

Children: 1 two to four times daily.
With the addition of a bronchodilator.

betamethasone   BEXTASOL   inhaler (100mcg/dose)
Initially 2 puffs four times daily reducing to minimum effective dose.
Same for adults and children.

budesonide   PULMICORT   inhaler (200mcg/dose)
1 puff twice daily. Severe cases up to 8 puffs daily.

                  PULMICORT LS   inhaler (50mcg/dose)
Children: 1–4 puffs twice daily.

                  PULMICORT   inhaler (200 or 400mcg/
                  TURBOHALER   dose)
200–1600mcg daily.
Children: 200–800mcg daily.

MAST CELL STABILISERS

These are often Category II but if the patient is very allergic then Category III would be more appropriate.

These are used in allergic conditions to prevent the release of histamine which is one of the main chemical mediators of the allergic reaction. Therefore, they are used prophylactically to prevent an attack and people are told to take them regularly. Although they are considered not to affect an acute attack it is people's experience that they do relieve wheezing at the time.

KETOTIFEN

Contraindications:
This drug is not to be given with oral hypoglycaemic agents.
Precautions:
There is an exacerbation of the asthma in 2/1000 cases.
Effects:
This drug also has antihistamine effects.
General: drowsiness, weight gain.
Central nervous system: dizziness.
Gastrointestinal: dry mouth.

CHEM NAME	TRADE NAME	FORMULATION
ketotifen	ZADITEN	1mg, 1mg/5ml

1–2mg twice daily.
Children: Under 2 years, not recommended. Over 2 years, 1mg twice daily.

SODIUM CROMOGLYCATE

Withdrawal in some patients who have severe problems which are allergic in nature may lead to the appearance of serious symptoms.

Effects:
These are considered to be minor when taken locally or inhaled such as throat irritation or coughing on inhalation. Severe bronchospasm and/or worsening of asthma is seen occasionally due to a hypersensitivity reaction.

General: muscle pain, joint pain and swelling, systemic lupus erythematosus syndrome.

Respiratory: pulmonary infiltration, pulmonary eosinophilia.

Gastrointestinal: gastroenteritis, nausea, oesophagitis.

Central nervous system: headache, dizziness.

Skin: dermatitis, pruritus.

CHEM NAME	TRADE NAME	FORMULATION
sodium cromoglycate	INTAL	spincaps (20mg/dose)

4 daily at regular intervals increasing if necessary to 6 or 8 daily.
Therapy should be continuous. Same dose for adults and children.

	INTAL 5	inhaler (5mg/dose)

Maintenance 1 puff four times daily.

	INTAL Compound	inhaler (20mg with isoprenaline 0.1mg/dose)

As INTAL SPINCAPS.
With the addition of a beta agonist.

NEDOCROMIL

This is a specific bronchial anti–inflammatory drug and is intended to be prophylactic and so should be taken regularly.

Effects:
Few are reported in the literature.

Central nervous system: headache.

Gastrointestinal: bitter taste in the mouth, nausea.

CHEM NAME	TRADE NAME	FORMULATION
nedocromil	TILADE	inhaler (2mg/dose)

2 puffs twice daily increasing if necessary to 2 puffs four times daily.
Children: not recommended.

COMMENTS

Asthma is very common and the mainstay of conventional treatment is by drugs. There is an emphasis these days on early diagnosis in children where there is a history of cough, maybe only at night, with wheezing. Many will be prescribed drugs usually in the inhaled form.

Inhaled drugs do cause less general side-effects than if they were taken orally but their effect on the lung tends to be more insidious and, of course, still suppressive. This effect is not particularly noticed unless people are compared with 'normals' or until the drug is reduced or stopped.

The first-line treatment is with a bronchodilator which stimulates the lungs and heart and so, long term, lead to weakness of these organs. Therefore, the longer patients have taken these drugs the more likely there is to be chronic damage. In fact bronchodilators in the past such as ephedrine and adrenaline have led to deaths. There is currently some belief, even in orthodox circles, that increasing asthma deaths now may be linked to these agents, particularly fenoterol. In recent months (1990) fenoterol has been withdrawn in New Zealand and Australia.

The prophylactic agents for allergic conditions are taken regularly and are considered not to be effective in an acute attack. This is not strictly true as I have seen several asthmatics who gain relief from wheezing by taking a dose of INTAL at the time of the attack. They would therefore seem to have similar energetic effects to the bronchodilators. They come somewhere between the corticosteroids and the bronchodilators in terms of severity of action. One problem with their use is that it is almost impossible to make a diagnosis while patients take them because the whole clinical picture is changed.

The emphasis should be to try to wean patients onto less powerful agents as treatment progresses. In that way alternative treatment will be antidoted less and less and the clinical picture will become more obvious.

Table of drugs in order of increasing strength:

CATEGORY I
- bronchodilator (symptomatic) — sympathomimetic; xanthine/beta agonist; anticholinergic

CATEGORY II
- bronchodilator (prophylactic) — sympathomimetic; xanthine/beta agonist; anticholinergic

CATEGORY II OR CATEGORY III

- mast cell inhibitor

CATEGORY III

- inhaled corticosteroids
- oral corticosteroids

Any corticosteroid should be withdrawn slowly because of its powerful suppressive action and the release of symptoms which may occur when it is reduced in dosage. If the patient is taking oral forms as say prednisolone then reduce by no more than 1mg each month. If the patient is taking 7mg per day which is quite a high dose it may well take up to a year to withdraw it.

It is quite in order for people to take more of their bronchodilator (within the limitations of the maximum dose) whilst this is happening because it will have less of a suppressant effect and will be less likely to antidote your treatment.

If working with a doctor then try to substitute an inhaled form for the oral whenever possible. Then reduce the inhaled corticosteroid.

When the steroid has been stopped, you can turn to the prophylactic agents such as INTAL or ZADITEN. Reduce these slowly also since there may well be a release of suppressed symptoms. The problems here will be less than with the corticosteroids.

If there is no suggestion of allergic disease, and some patients notice no or very little benefit from INTAL and the like, then stop it at the very beginning of drug management.

Finally, the bronchodilator should be attended to. I always try to encourage people to try and use it only when necessary and then only after trying to deal with the wheezing situation in some other way such as by rest or by relaxation. Unless the wheezing is very severe there is no harm in allowing a wheeze to subside on its own with rest or relaxation.

Indications of a severe case or attack of asthma would be indicated by rapid pulse rate (>120), cyanosis, severe breathlessness even at rest or with minimal exercise, frequent use of inhalers with little relief and eventually mental symptoms such as confusion. Appearance of any of these necessitates emergency treatment of the acute attack.

9   GASTROINTESTINAL SYSTEM

NAUSEA, VOMITING

Many of these drugs may be used for balance disorders such as dizziness, vertigo, Meniere's disease as well as nausea or vomiting of gastrointestinal origin.

They are often powerful drugs with effects in the central nervous system. They may be used in mild cases.

HISTAMINE ANALOGUE

Category II drug.
Contraindications:
Phaeochromocytoma.
Precautions:
Bronchial asthma and peptic ulcer.
Effects:
Gastrointestinal: nausea, vomiting, indigestion.
Central nervous system: headache.
Skin: flushing.

CHEM NAME	TRADE NAME	FORMULATION
betahistine	SERC	8mg
Maintenance 3–6 daily.		

ANTIHISTAMINE

Category II drug unless the patient is very allergic in which case it may be more appropriate to consider in Category III. These are mainly used in cases of allergic disease and are described in detail on page 151.

This group of drugs is used widely for nausea and vomiting, allergic reactions such as urticaria, hay fever.

Some are used also for the treatment of motion sickness.

CHEM NAME	TRADE NAME	FORMULATION
cinnarizine	STUGERON	15mg

Inner ear disorders: 2 three times daily.
Motion sickness, 2 two hours before, then 1 eight hourly during journey.
Children: under 5 years not recommended, 5–12 years half adult dose.

cyclizine   VALOID   50mg
50mg three times daily.
Children: under 1 year not recommended, 1–10 years 25mg, 10–12
years 50mg. Both three times daily.

dimenhydrinate   DRAMAMINE   50mg
1–2 two or three times daily.
Children: under 1 year not recommended, 1–6 years quarter to half a
tablet, 7–12 years half to 1 tablet. Both two or three times daily.

promethazine   AVOMINE   25mg
Motion sickness, 1 at bedtime before long journey or 1–2 hours before
short journeys.
Nausea, 1 once to three times daily.
Children: under 5 years not recommended, 5–10 years half adult dose.

ANTICHOLINERGIC

Category II drug.
These are also used in the treatment of asthma and diarrhoea.
See page 151 for details.

CHEM NAME	TRADE NAME	FORMULATION
hyoscine	SCOPODERM	1.5mg adhesive patch

For motion sickness. 1–2 patches applied during journey — interval of
72 hours. Same dose for children over 10 years.

DOPAMINE ANTAGONISTS

Category II drug.
This group of drugs acts through the central nervous system
and explains why most of its effects, particularly the severe
ones, occur in this area.

CHEM NAME	TRADE NAME	FORMULATION
domperidone	EVOXIN	10mg, 30mg suppositories
	MOTILIUM	10mg, 1mg/ml, 30mg suppositories

1–2 tablets or 2 suppositories four to eight hourly.
This drug has some similarities with metoclopramide (see below) but
the extrapyramidal effects are less frequent. It may also cause gynaecomastia and galactorrhoea.

METOCLOPRAMIDE

Category II drug.

This drug is related to the antipsychotic drugs and there are some similarities in its effects.

Precautions:

Epilepsy, cases where other drugs are taken which act on the central nervous system, renal impairment.

Parkinsonian symptoms of rigidity, tremor and slow movement may occur with this drug and antipsychotic agents so caution when both are prescribed.

Effects:

General: drowsiness.

Gastrointestinal: diarrhoea.

Central nervous system: dyskinesia, spasms of the facial muscles, trismus, rhythmic protrusion of the tongue, spasm of the ocular muscles, unnatural positioning of the head and shoulders and opisthotonos. There may be generalised increase in muscle tone. Tardive dyskinesia has occurred with long-term treatment particularly in the elderly. Parkinsonism.

Psychological: restlessness.

CHEM NAME	TRADE NAME	FORMULATION
metoclopramide	GASTRESE LA	15mg continous-release
	GASTROBID CONTINUS	15mg sustained-release
	GASTROFLUX	10mg
	GASTROMAX	30mg sustained-release
	MAXOLON SR	15mg sustained-release

Over 20 years, 30mg daily. Usual maximum 0.5mg/Kg body-weight daily.

Children: not recommended.

	MAXOLON	10mg, 5mg/5ml, 1mg/ml
	METOX	10mg
	PARMID	10mg, 5mg/5ml
	PRIMPERAN	10mg, 5mg/5ml

Adults of 20 years and over: 10mg three times daily.

Children: only for severe, intractable nausea and vomiting of known cause and vomiting associated with cytotoxic drugs and radiotherapy.

PHENOTHIAZINE

Category II drug here although in higher doses for psychoses it would be in Category IV.

Prochlorperazine particularly is commonly used to treat nausea and vomiting and included in this same group is the antipsychotic agent LARGACTIL. See page 93 for details).

CHEM NAME	TRADE NAME	FORMULATION
pro-chlorperazine	BUCCASTEM	3mg

1–2 twice daily. Leave to dissolve between upper lip and gum.
Not for children.

	STEMETIL	5mg, 5mg and 25mg suppositories 5mg/5ml

Vertigo, 5mg three times daily. Maximum 30mg daily.
Nausea and vomiting: prophylaxis 5–10mg two or three times daily.
Suppositories: 25mg then oral medication if required.
Children: under 10Kg not recommended, over 10Kg 0.25mg/Kg two or three times daily.

	VERTIGON SPANSULE	10mg, 15mg both sustained-release

Maintenance 10–15mg daily.
Not for children.

thiethyl-perazine	TORECAN	6.33mg, 6.5mg suppository

1 two or three times daily.
Suppository: 1 night and evening.
Not for children.

trifluoperazine	STELAZINE	1mg, 2mg

2–6mg daily.
Children: under 3 years not recommended, 3–5 years up to 1mg daily, 6–12 years up to 4 mg daily.

Peptic Ulcer, Dyspepsia

There are many remedies for upper abdominal discomfort and pain which are available over-the-counter and as prescribed drugs. There are two main groups — those used to neutralise acid and those which have specific anti-ulcer properties. The latter type include the newer drugs such as TAGAMET and ZANTAC.

These were originally given only in cases of proven peptic ulcers but in recent years, and increasingly so, they are also given in cases where either there is no ulcer seen on investigation or even without any investigation performed. This use of powerful drugs for simple indigestion is often inappropriate and presents more problems for alternative practitioners.

ANTACID

Category I if taken symptomatcally or Category II if taken regularly.

There are many types of agent taken to neutralise gastric acidity and relieve indigestion. They are symptomatic in nature and do nothing to change the underlying pathology. With continued use they actually lead to the production of more gastric acid as the stomach tries to maintain an acidic pH. So the taking of these drugs tends to be self-perpetuating unless treatment is aimed at the cause.

Most antacid preparations contain either aluminium, magnesium or a combination. Aluminium has been implicated in the development of certain types of dementia and certainly high blood levels may cause encephalopathy in the short term. It also causes constipation.

Magnesium leads to diarrhoea and loose stools.

Sodium salts may affect patients with heart disease to precipitate or aggravate cardiac failure.

Large doses of antacids may cause the milk-alkali syndrome which is an acute onset of headache, nausea, irritability and weakness.

All antacids may affect the absorption of drugs and some contain enough sugar to affect diabetic control.

CHEM NAME	TRADE NAME	FORMULATION
almasilate	MALINAL	500mg/5ml
10ml at meal times and bedtime.		
aluminium hydroxide	ALU-CAP	475mg
	ACTONORM GEL	220mg with magnesium hydroxide, dimethicone
5–20ml after meals.		
With the addition of a deflatulent.		
	ALGICON	360mg with magnesium alginate, magnesium carbonate, potassium bicarbonate

1–2 tablets or 10–20ml suspension four times daily.
1 four times daily and bedtime.
With the addition of a reflux suppressant.

ALUDROX — gel

5–10ml four times daily.

ALUDROX SA — with ambutonium bromide, magnesium hydroxide

5–10ml three or four times daily.
With the addition of an anticholinergic agent.

ALUHYDE — 245mg with magnesium trisilicate, belladonna liq. extract

2 after meals.
With the addition of an anticholinergic agent.

ANDURSIL — 200mg with magnesium hydroxide, aluminium hydroxide/ magnesium carbonate combined, dimethicone

5–10ml or 1–2 tablets three or four times daily.
With the addition of other antacids and a deflatulent.

APP — with papaverine, homatropine, calcium carbonate, magnesium carbonate, magnesium trisilicate, bismuth carbonate

5ml or 1–2 tablets three or four times daily.
With the addition of antispasmodics, anticholinergic and other antacids.

ASILONE — 420mg with dimethicone, magnesium oxide

5–10ml or 1–2 tablets before meals and at bedtime.
With the addition of a deflatulent.

CAVED-S — 100mg with deglycyrrhinized licorice, magnesium carbonate, sodium bicarbonate

2 chewed three to six times daily.
With the addition of a specific antiulcer agent (licorice).

DIOVOL — 200mg with magnesium hydroxide, dimethicone

5–10ml as required.
With the addition of a deflatulent.

GELUSIL — 250mg with magnesium trisilicate

1–2 tablets when required.

KOLANTICON   400mg with magnesium
oxide, dicyclomine,
dimethicone

10–20ml four hourly.
With the addition of an anticholinergic agent and a deflatulent.

MAALOX   220mg with magnesium
hydroxide

10–20ml or 1–2 tablets four times daily.

MAALOX PLUS   220mg with magnesium
hydroxide, dimethicone

1–2 tablets or 5–10ml suspension four times daily.
With the addition of a deflatulent.

MAALOX TC   with magnesium
hydroxide

3 tablets or 15ml twice daily.

MUCAINE   with oxethazine,
magnesium hydroxide

5–10ml three or four times daily.
With the addition of a local anaesthetic.

MUCOGEL   with magnesium
hydroxide

10–20ml or 1–2 tablets three times daily.

POLYCROL Forte   with dimethicone,
magnesium hydroxide

1–2 tablets or 5–10ml four times daily.
With the addition of a deflatulent.

POLYCROL   as above but less
dimethicone

1–2 tablets or 5–10ml four times daily.
With the addition of a deflatulent.

SILOXYL   with dimethicone

1–2 tablets or 5–10ml four times daily.
With the addition of a deflatulent.

SIMECO   with magnesium
hydroxide, dimethicone

1–2 tablets or 5–10ml four times daily.
With the addition of a deflatulent.

UNIGEST   with dimethicone

1–2 tablets four times daily.
With the addition of a deflatulent.

calcium carbonate   NULACIN   130mg with whole milk
solids, magnesium
trisilicate, magnesium
oxide, magnesium

carbonate

1 or more as required.

	RABRO	500mg with licorice, magnesium oxide, frangula

1–2 three times daily.
With the addition of a specific antiulcer agent (licorice) and a bulking agent (frangula).

hydrotalcite	ALTACITE ALTACITE PLUS	500mg, 500mg/5ml with dimethicone

10ml or 2 tablets four times daily.
With the addition of a deflatulent.

magaldrate	DYNESE	800mg/5ml

5–10ml four times daily.

magnesium carbonate	ROTER	with bismuth subnitrate, sodium bicarbonate, frangula

1–2 three times daily.
With the addition of a specific antiulcer agent (bismuth) and a bulking agent (frangula).

magnesium hydroxide	MAGNESIUM HYDROXIDE MIXTURE	

5–10ml as required.

magnesium trisilicate	MAGNESIUM TRISILICATE MIXTURE	

10–20ml or 1–2 tablets as necessary.

sodium bicarbonate	SODIUM BICARBONATE TABLETS CO.	300mg with peppermint oil

2–6 tablets as required.
With the addition of an antispasmodic.

REFLUX SUPPRESSANT

Category II drugs.
The aim of this is to reduce reflux of acid up into the oesophagus and is therefore used in cases of reflux oesophagitis.

CHEM NAME	TRADE NAME	FORMULATION
alginic acid	GASTROCOTE	200mg with aluminium hydroxide, magnesium trisilicate, sodium bicarbonate

1 or 2 tablets or 5–15ml four times daily and at bedtime.

With the addition of antacids.

GASTRON		600mg with sodium bicarbonate, magnesium trisilicate

With the addition of antacids.

GAVISCON		500mg with magnesium trisilicate, aluminium hydroxide, sodium bicarbonate

1 or 2 tablets or 10–20ml after meals and at night.
With the addition of antacids.

TOPAL		200mg with aluminium hydroxide, magnesium carbonate

1–3 chewed three or four times daily.
With the addition of antacids.

ANTISPASMODIC

Category II drug.
There are varying examples of this group of drugs. There are very few effects written in the literature.

CHEM NAME	TRADE NAME	FORMULATION
alverine citrate	SPASMONAL	60mg

1–2 one to three times daily.

mebeverine	COLOFAC	135mg, 50mg/5ml

1 tablet or 15ml three times daily.

	COLVEN	with ispaghula husk

1 sachet twice or three times daily.
With the addition of a bulking agent.

PEPPERMINT OIL

Category II drug.
Precautions:
Breaking the capsules in the mouth may lead to irritation of the mouth or oesophagus.

Effects:
Cardiovascular: slow pulse rate.
Central nervous system: muscle tremor, headache, ataxia.
Gastrointestinal: heartburn.
Allergy: sensitivity reactions.
Skin: rashes.
Withdrawal may lead to abdominal cramps, distension and bowel disturbances.

CHEM NAME	TRADE NAME	FORMULATION
peppermint oil	COLPERMIN	0.2ml
	MINTEC	0.2ml

1–2 three times daily. Maximum 2 three times daily.

ANTICHOLINERGIC

Category II drug.
These drugs are also used in asthma and diarrhoea. See page 173 for full details.

CHEM NAME	TRADE NAME	FORMULATION
belladonna	BELLOCARB	10mg with magnesium trisilicate, magnesium carbonate

1–2 four times daily.
With the addition of antacids.

	CARBELLON	6mg with magnesium hydroxide, charcoal, peppermint oil

2–4 three times daily.
With the addition of an antacid and an antispasmodic.

dicyclomine	MERBENTYL	10mg, 20mg, 10mg/5ml

10–20mg three times daily.
Children: up to 6 months not recommended, 6 months–2 years 5–10mg three or four times daily (maximum 40mg daily), over 2 years 10mg three times daily.

hyoscine	BUSCOPAN	10mg

2 four times daily.
Children: under 6 years not recommended, 6–12 years 1 three times daily.
This drug is also used in the treatment of 'spasmodic' dysmenorrhoea. It is given in the dose above (for adults) from 2 days

before menstruation until 3 days into the period.

mepenozalate   CANTIL   25mg, 12.5mg/5ml
1–2 tablets or 10–20ml three or four times daily.
Children: under 6 years not recommended, 6–12 years 5ml three or
four times daily.

pipenozalate   PIPTAL   5mg
1 three times daily and 1–2 at night.
Not for children.

PIPTALIN   4mg with dimethicone
(40mg)/5ml
10ml three or four times daily.
Children: up to 10Kg 2.5ml, 10–20Kg 2.5–5ml, 20–40Kg 5ml. All three
or four times daily.
With the addition of a deflatulent.

pirenzepine   GASTROZEPIN   50mg
1 twice daily for 4–6 weeks.

propantheline   PRO–BANTHINE   15mg
Ulcer, initially 1 three times daily and two at bedtime. Other indications, up to 8 daily.

poldine   NACTON FORTE   4mg
1 four times daily.

NACTON   2mg
1 four times daily. Used in the elderly when a lower dosage required.
Dosage is increased until dry mouth, blurred vision or urinary
hesitancy appears then dosage is reduced slightly!

H2 BLOCKER

Category II drug.
This group of drugs has revolutionised the conventional treatment of peptic ulcers since they were first introduced about 12
years ago. They are also widely used for all types of upper
abdominal gastrointestinal pain and dyspepsia. They act by
preventing the stomach producing normal amounts of gastric
acid.
Precautions:
Treatment with these drugs may mask and temporarily heal
gastric carcinoma and so diagnosis may be delayed.
Effects:
General: tiredness, myalgia, arthralgia.
Cardiovascular: rapid pulse rate, slow pulse rate, palpitations.

Gastrointestinal: nausea, diarrhoea, liver damage, pancreatitis, cancer of the stomach.

Central nervous system: dizziness, headache, extrapyramidal effects.

Psychological: confusional states. This is seen more with cimetidine than the others.

Endocrine: gynaecomastia.

Urogenital: nephritis, impotence, reduced sperm counts.

Blood: aplastic anaemia, thrombocytopenia.

Skin: rash, alopecia.

CHEM NAME	TRADE NAME	FORMULATION
cimetidine	DYSPAMET	200mg, 200mg/5ml
	TAGAMET	200mg, 400mg, 800mg

Duodenal ulcer — 800mg bedtime or 400mg twice daily for minimum of 4 weeks.
Maintenance 400mg bedtime or twice daily.

	ALGITEC	200mg with 500mg alginic acid

1–2 tablets four times a day for four to eight weeks.
With the addition of a reflux suppressant.

famotidine	PEPCID PM	20mg, 40mg

40mg at night for 4–8 weeks. Prophylaxis of relapse — 20mg at night.

nizatidine	AXID	150mg, 300mg

300mg daily for four to eight weeks. Prophylaxis: 150mg daily for up to a year.

ranitidine	ZANTAC	150mg, 300mg, 150mg/10ml

For duodenal and gastric ulceration, 150mg twice daily or 300mg at night for four weeks.
Maintenance 150mg at night.

PROKINETIC

Category II drug.

This is a new type of drug which stimulates the gastrointestinal musculature to produce more rapid transit of contents through the system. Its exact mode of action at the biochemical level is unclear.

Contraindications:

The drug should not be used in those where gastrointestinal stimulation is dangerous, i.e. gastrointestinal haemorrhage, obstruction or perforation.

Precautions:
The main problems are with concurrent administration of drugs such as benzodiazepines and alcohol (increased sedation) and anticonvulsants where blood levels may have to be monitored. The drug leads to reduced gastric absorption and increased small intestine absorption and this is important when considering interactions with other drugs which may be absorbed in one or other sites.

Effects:
General: sleepiness, fatigue.
Central nervous system: headache, lightheadedness, convulsions.
Gastrointestinal: borborygmi, flatus, diarrhoea.
Urogenital: urinary frequency.

CHEM NAME	TRADE NAME	FORMULATION
cisapride	ALIMIX	10mg
	PREPULSID	10mg

1 three or four times daily for 3 months. For oesophageal reflux.

PROSTAGLANDIN ANALOGUE

Category II drug.
These are very new drugs with little available information.
Precautions:
Cases where low blood pressure may be a problem such as cerebrovascular disease, coronary artery disease, severe peripheral vascular disease or hypertension.

Effects:
Gastrointestinal: diarrhoea in 10% of patients, abdominal pain, dyspepsia, flatulence, nausea.
Urogenital: abnormal vaginal bleeding — intermenstrual bleeding, menorrhagia, post-menopausal bleeding.

CHEM NAME	TRADE NAME	FORMULATION
misoprostol	CYTOTEC	200mcg

4 daily for 4–8 weeks.
Prophylaxis, 1 tablet two to four times daily whilst taking drugs such anti-inflammatory drugs for arthritis which have a propensity for causing indigestion.

PROTON PUMP INHIBITOR

Category II drug.

This is new range of drugs very different from others aimed at gastric disorders. It will almost certainly herald the production of related chemicals cashing in on the expected response. Its action is to reduce the production of gastric acid.

Contraindications:

None known.

Precautions:

The diagnosis of gastric carcinoma may be delayed because this drug, as with ZANTAC et al, may improve the symptoms of this condition.

Effects:

Central nervous system: headache.

Gastrointestinal: nausea, diarrhoea, constipation, flatulence.

Skin: rash.

CHEM NAME	TRADE NAME	FORMULATION
meprazole	LOSEC	20mg
1–2 daily. NOT for long term use.		

CYTOPROTECTANT

Category II drug.

This group of drugs has specific antiulcer actions. They are the older types of remedy and tend to be less powerful than the more modern H2 blockers. Their effects therefore are less hazardous.

CARBENOLOXONE

This tends to lead to sodium and water retention. It is more a problem in the elderly or in hepatic and renal impairment where this may have an effect on hypertension and cardiac failure. Potassium loss also occurs and this may lead to symptoms such as weakness, tiredness, frequent urination. See diuretics on page 118 for details.

CHEM NAME	TRADE NAME	FORMULATION
carbenoxolone	BIOGASTRONE	50mg

1 three times daily until the ulcer is healed (usually 4–6 weeks but may be 12 weeks). For gastric ulcer.

	DUOGASTRONE	50mg

1 four times daily for 6–12 weeks. For duodenal ulcer.

	PYROGASTRONE	20mg with magnesium trisilicate, aluminium hydroxide, sodium alginate, potassium bicarbonate

1 tablet or 10ml three times daily after meals and two tablets or 20ml at bedtime. For oesophagitis.
With the addition of antacids and a reflux suppressant.

SUCRALFATE

Category II drug.
Precautions:
It should be used with caution in those with renal impairment.
Effects:
This drug may lead to an accumulation of aluminium.
General: back pain, sleeplessness.
Central nervous system: dizziness, vertigo.
Gastrointestinal: diarrhoea, nausea, gastric discomfort, indigestion, dry mouth.
Skin: rash, itching.

CHEM NAME	TRADE NAME	FORMULATION
sucralfate	ANTEPSIN	1G

2 twice daily for at least four weeks.

BISMUTH COMPOUNDS

Category II drug.
Contraindications:
Renal disorders.
Effects:
Gastrointestinal: blackening of the stool, darkening of the tongue occur due to discolouring effects, nausea, vomiting.

Central nervous system: speech disorder, ataxia.
Psychological: confusion.

CHEM NAME	TRADE NAME	FORMULATION
tripotassium dicitrato bismuthate	DE-NOL	120mg/5ml

10ml twice daily. Continue for 28 or 56 days as necessary.

	DE-NOLTAB	120mg

2 tablets twice daily. Continue for 28 or 56 days as necessary.

COMMENTS

When dealing with upper abdominal problems such as indigestion or even peptic ulcer remember that most remedies are used for symptomatic relief. Only the H2 blockers, the cytoprotectants and newer drugs such as CYTOTEC and LOSEC actually try to do anything about the ulcer itself.

When H2 blockers are given they very quickly relieve the symptoms of peptic ulceration or indigestion. They are powerful suppressive agents. However, when they are stopped they may lead to a rebound appearance of these same symptoms even after several years.

It has been recognised for a long time that maintenance therapy is needed in many cases of a reduced dosage at night. Even if the drug was originally used for gastrointestinal haemorrhage there may be a recurrence when the drug is finally stopped.

There is some evidence that long-term use of these drugs may actually lead to the development of gastric carcinoma. It is well known that this condition is related to conditions of low or absent gastric acid. These drugs produce such a state.

Table of drugs in order of increasing strength:

CATEGORY I
- antacid (symptomatic)

CATEGORY II
- antacid (prophylactic)
- antispasmodic
- cytoprotectant
- anticholinergic
- H2 blockers

Reduction of antiulcer drugs can lead to reappearance of the original symptom picture and must be done slowly in conjunction with your treatment.

Once this has been achieved then move onto the antacid. The frequent use of antacids actually leads to the secretion of INCREASED levels of acid as the stomach tries to maintain a normal level of pH. If reduction of the antacid is too rapid then the upper gastrointestinal tract will be exposed to the full force of this increased acid level.

The removal of other factors which tend to lead to increases in acid such as cigarettes, coffee, acid food and spices will all help in this process.

Bowel disorders in general often respond well to alternative medicine and once the more powerful antiulcer drugs have been removed progress should be more rapid.

Iron Preparations

These are all to be considered as Category I drugs since they are given symptomatically for the treatment of iron deficiency. They cause no problems on withdrawal.

These drugs are used to treat iron deficiency problems such as anaemia. They may also be used in patients with debility, tiredness and anaemias which are not of an iron deficiency type.

They are very irritative and commonly lead to symptoms in the gastrointestinal tract such as constipation, nausea and vomiting.

There are much better ways of replacing iron such as through diet, using herbs to strengthen blood and so on. I invariably tell people to stop them. Sudden withdrawal is not a problem.

Patients with anaemia may usefully have their haemoglobin monitored so that treatment is seen to be effective.

Remember that not all anaemias are due to a deficiency of iron.

Effects:

Gastrointestinal: dark stools, anorexia, vomiting, nausea, abdominal discomfort, constipation, diarrhoea. These are reduced if taken with food.

Allergic reactions.

Zinc may lead to nausea.

CHEM NAME	TRADE NAME	FORMULATION
ferric citrate	LEXPEC WITH IRON	with folic acid
	LEXPEC WITH IRON-M	with folic acid
ferrous fumarate	B.C.500 with Iron	with vitamins B and C
	FERROCAP	
	FERROCAP-F 350	with folic acid
	FERSADAY	
	FERSAMAL	
	FOLEX-350	with folic acid
	GALFER	
	GALFER F.A.	with folic acid
	GALFERVIT	with vitamins B and C
	GIVITOL	with vitamins B and C
	METERFOLIC	with folic acid
	PREGADAY	with folic acid
ferrous gluconate	FERFOLIC SV	with folic acid
	FERGON	
ferrous sulphate	FEFOL SPANSULE	with folic acid,
	FEFOL-VIT SPANSULE	with folic acid, vitamins B and C
	FEFOL Z SPANSULE	with folic acid, zinc
	FEOSPAN SPANSULE	
	FERROCONTIN CONTINUS	
	FERROCONTIN FOLIC CONTINUS	with folic acid
	FERROGRAD	
	FERROGRAD C	with vitamin C
	FERROGRAD FOLIC	with folic acid
	FESOVIT SPANSULE	with vitamin B and C
	FESOVIT Z SPANSULE	with vitamin B and C, zinc
	FOLICIN	with folic acid, copper, manganese
	PLESMET	
	PREGNAVITE Forte F	with folic acid, vitamins B, C, D
SLOW-FE		
SLOW-FE Folic		with folic acid
ferrous succinate	FERROMYN	
iron complex	NIFEREX	
	SYTRON	

Laxatives

These are in Category I if taken on an occasional basis and Category II if taken regularly.

They are used in the treatment of constipation. Although such drugs are better reserved for occasional use only there are many instances where regular use is seen. This is also true for related compounds available over-the-counter.

Habitual use of laxatives leads to weak bowel musculature and eventually constipation. Weaning patients off these can be very difficult and is a slow process as the bowel has to relearn how to function unaided. Diet clearly plays an important part here.

STIMULANT

There are varying types, all have similar effects.
Contraindications:
Undiagnosed acute or persistent abdominal symptoms.
Effects:
Temporary griping pains in the abdomen.

CHEM NAME	TRADE NAME	FORMULATION
aloin	ALOPHEN	15mg with phenolphthalein, ipecacuanha, belladonna

1–3 at bedtime.
With the addition of an anticholinergic agent.

bisacodyl	DULCOLAX	5mg, suppositories 5mg and 10mg

2 tablets at night or 1x10mg suppository morning.

danthron	CODALAX	25mg with poloxamer

5–10ml at night.
With the addition of a faecal softener.

	CODALAX FORTE	75mg with poloxamer

2.5–5ml at night.
With the addition of a faecal softener.

	CO-DANTHRUSATE	50mg with 60mg docusate sodium
	NORMAX	50mg with 60mg docusate sodium

1–3 at night when required.

With the addition of a faecal softener.

sennosides	SENNA TABLETS	7.5mg
2–4 at bedtime.		
	SENOKOT	7.5mg, granules 15mg/5ml, syrup 15mg/10ml
2–4 tablets or 5–10ml granules or 10–20ml syrup bedtime.		
sodium picosulphate	LAXOBERAL	5mg/5ml
	SODIUM PICOSULPHATE	5mg/5ml
5–15ml nocte.		

BULKING AGENT

There are several types based upon different types of fibre. Some may also be used in the treatment of obesity, diarrhoea and to control appetite.
Contraindications:
Diarrhoea caused by infection or bowel obstruction.
Effects:
There are none listed.
You would expect them to lead to problems of wind, distension and abdominal discomfort in susceptible individuals.
Their sugar content may affect diabetic control.

CHEM NAME	TRADE NAME	FORMULATION
bran	FYBRANTA	2G bran
1–3 three or four times daily.		
	LEJFIBRE	4.04G oat bran meal biscuit
2 daily.		
grain fibre	PROCTOFIBE	375mg with citrus fibre
4–12 daily.		
ispaghula husk	FYBOGEL	3.5G sachets
1 sachet twice daily.		
	ISOGEL	Granules
10ml once or twice daily.		
	MANEVAC	with sennosides
5–10ml at night and if necessary morning.		

Obstinate cases, 10ml 6 hourly for up to 3 days.
With the addition of a stimulant.

	REGULAN	3.6G sachets

1 sachet one to three times daily.

methylcellulose	CELEVAC	500mg

3–6 tablets twice daily.

	COLOGEL	450mg/5ml

5–15ml three times daily.

sterculia	NORMACOL	

1–2 sachets or 1–2 heaped 5ml spoonfuls once or twice daily.

	NORMACOL PLUS	with frangula

1–2 sachets or 1–2 heaped 5ml spoonfuls once or twice daily.
With the addition of another bulking agent.

FAECAL SOFTENER
Contraindications:
Abdominal pain, nausea or vomiting, at the same time as mineral oil or to those under 6 months of age.
Effects:
There are none listed.

CHEM NAME	TRADE NAME	FORMULATION
docusate sodium	DIOCTYL	100mg, 50mg/5ml

Up to 500mg daily.

	DIOCTYL PAEDIATRIC SYRUP	12.5mg/5ml

12.5–25mg three times daily.

LUBRICANT

This merely acts to lubricate the intestines and there is a possible risk of inhalation with subsequent pneumonia. It may also interfere with the absorption of fat soluble vitamins.

CHEM NAME	TRADE NAME	FORMULATION
liquid paraffin	AGAROL	with phenolphthalein, agar

5–15ml bedtime.
With the addition of a stimulant.

	PETROLAGAR No1	

10ml twice daily.

OSMOTIC LAXATIVE

These are effective by drawing fluid out of the body to soften the faeces.

LACTULOSE
Contraindications:
Galactosaemia or where there is evidence of gastrointestinal obstruction.
Precautions:
Lactose intolerance.
Effects:
Gastrointestinal: abdominal distension, flatulence, diarrhoea.

CHEM NAME	TRADE NAME	FORMULATION
lactulose	DUPHALAC	3.35G/5ml
Initially 15ml twice daily.		
magnesium sulphate	MAGNESIUM SULPHATE MIXTURE	
10–20ml.		
	MAGNESIUM SULPHATE CRYSTALS	
5–15G when required.		
	KEST	with phenolphthalein
1 at night, two morning.		
With the addition of a stimulant.		
sodium bicarbonate	CARBALAX	1.08G with sodium acid phosphate (suppository)
1 suppository 30 minutes before evacuation required.		

COMMENTS

Most agents listed here are prescribed in the belief that the bowel needs to be stimulated or the faeces are too hard. So either bran/fibre supplements are taken or chemicals which directly affect the bowel musculature.
Stimulants weaken the bowel and eventually it fails to work at all without the drugs.
If they are taken infrequently for occasional constipation there will be few problems for the practitioner. View them as for any symptomatic drug.

When regular medication occurs this is more difficult. Gradual reduction needs to be followed by treatment and time to allow the bowel to recover its function.

I once treated a woman who took 24 SENOKOT each day! She was only 26 years of age and her constipation began after a hysterectomy at the age of 23. Her bowel was severely weakened by the dose of senna. This is an exceptional case in terms of dosage but many people take laxatives on an occasional or more frequent basis.

Purgative abuse, as it is known, is commonest with stimulants. It can lead to chronic diarrhoea and thence thirst, tiredness, weight loss, oedema and bone pain because of loss of electrolytes.

Antidiarrhoeals

Diarrhoea is very common and can be usefully be divided into acute and chronic cases. The acute types tend to be due either to infection or dietary indiscretion. They usually subside on their own and the major problem is in young babies where dehydration may develop.

The chronic forms are due to bowel disease such as Crohn's disease, ulcerative colitis, or perhaps as part of diverticulitis or as a symptom of cancer. Treatment of the symptom by drugs alone is potentially dangerous since it can mask the true diagnosis and does nothing to alleviate the underlying condition.

ABSORBENT

Category II drugs.

These merely have effects on drying the faeces. They are generally safe.

CHEM NAME	TRADE NAME	FORMULATION
ceratonia	AROBON	with starch

Adults and children: 20–40G in water daily.
Infants: 2–5G per 100ml feed.

kaolin	KAOPECTATE	1.03G/5ml

10–30ml every four hours.
Children: under 1 year 5ml, 1–5 years 10ml, over 5 years 10–30ml. All every four hours.

methylcellulose	CELEVAC	500mg

3–6 twice daily.

Children: in proportion to dosage for 70Kg adult.

OPIATE

Category II drugs but the most powerful in this section. These are commonly used as analgesics and are described in more detail on page 213. They have a constipating action which here is desirable but as an analgesic is considered to be a 'side-effect'.

CHEM NAME	TRADE NAME	FORMULATION
codeine phosphate	DIARREST	5mg with dicyclomine, potassium chloride, sodium chloride, sodium citrate/5ml

20ml four times daily.
Children: under 4 years only in special circumstances, 4–5 years 5ml, 6–9 years 10ml, 10–13 years 15ml. All four times daily.
With the addition of an anticholinergic and electrolytes.

	KAODENE	10mg with kaolin/10ml

20ml three or four times daily.
Children: under 5 years not recommended, over 5 years half the adult dose.
With the addition of an absorbent.

diphenoxylate	LOMOTIL	2.5mg with atropine (5ml liquid = 1 tablet)

4 tablets or 20ml initially then two tablets or 10ml six hourly until under control.
Children: under 4 years not recommended, 4–8 years one tablet or 5ml three times daily, 9–12 years one tablet or 5ml four times daily, 13–16 years two tablets or 10ml three times daily.
With the addition of an anticholinergic agent.
Children are especially sensitive to the opiate and/or anticholinergic effects of this drug.

loperamide	IMODIUM	2mg, 1mg/5ml

Acute diarrhoea: initially two then one at each loose stool (usually 3–4 daily). Maximum 8 daily.
Chronic diarrhoea: initially 2–4 daily.
Children: acute: under 4 not recommended, 4–8 years 5ml, 9–12 years one tablet or 10ml. Both four times daily.
This drug is generally safe but may cause nausea, dizziness, abdominal pain and dry mouth.

ELECTROLYTE

Category I.

These are given to replace salt and fluid lost because of the diarrhoea.

They can be life-saving in cases of dehydration especially in babies and infants.

Low sodium in the formulations may lead to low sodium levels in the patient. The sugar in some may cause diarrhoea.

CHEM NAME	TRADE NAME	FORMULATION
sodium chloride	DIORYLATE	with potassium chloride, sodium bicarbonate, glucose (sachets)
	ELECTROLADE	with potassium chloride, sodium bicarbonate, glucose, saccharine
	GLUCO-LYTE	with potassium chloride, sodium bicarbonate, glucose (sachets)
	REHIDRAT	with potassium chloride, sodium bicarbonate, glucose, citric acid, sucrose, laevulose

Adults and children: 1 or 2 after each loose motion.

Infants: reconstitute and substitute in equivalent volume to feeds.

COMMENTS

Drugs used here for diarrhoea are only ever symptomatic in that they are used to remove that symptom rather than treat the underlying condition.

Electrolyte replacement solutions are very useful to treat and prevent dehydration particularly in babies and infants. They have an important role to play in developing countries where loss of fluid from diarrhoea is a major cause of death. The formulation of such substances in packets produced by the pharmaceutical industry must be a very expensive way of providing them however.

The remainder act on the bowel primarily by slowing transit time. Opiates (morphine derivatives), anticholinergics and antispasmodics act on the bowel wall to reduce its action. This, of course, is quite harmful since it prevents the body from eliminating in the manner it requires.

Withdrawal of the drug may lead to diarrhoea, loose motions, colicky abdominal pains. Treatment should be directed at the cause rather the result.

The use of opiates long term may also lead to psychological symptoms because of their sedative actions. There may be the appearance of anxiety, restlessness and insomnia when withdrawn.

Colon/Rectum

These drugs are used for the treatment of local disease of the anus, rectum and colon such as haemorrhoids, colitis, anal fissure.

SOOTHING

Category II drugs.

CHEM NAME	TRADE NAME	FORMULATION
bismuth subgallate	ANUSOL	with bismuth oxide, Peru balsam, zinc oxide (cream, ointment and suppositories)

With the addition of antiseptics and astringents.

ANTI-INFLAMMATORY

CHEM NAME	TRADE NAME	FORMULATION
heparinoid	LASONIL	with hyaluronidase (ointment)

SALICYLATE

Category II drug.

A relation of aspirin. This group is used in the treatment of ulcerative colitis — to produce a remission and for maintenance.

Contraindications:
Severe renal impairment.
Precautions:
Renal impairment.
Effects:
Central nervous system: headache.
Gastrointestinal: nausea, diarrhoea, abdominal pain, exacerbation of colitis, pancreatitis.
Blood disorders: bone marrow depression.
Urogenital: depression of sperm count and sperm function.

CHEM NAME	TRADE NAME	FORMULATION
mesalazine	ASACOL	400mg
Maintenance 3–6 daily.		
	PENTASA	1G enema
1 at night.		
olsalazine	DIPENTUM	250mg
Maintenance 2 twice daily.		

SALICYLATE-SULPHONAMIDE

Category II drug.
A commonly used drug in ulcerative colitis. It is related to aspirin and the sulphonamide group of antibiotics.
Contraindications:
Infants under the age of 2 years.
Precautions:
Full blood counts should be performed before treatment begins and at monthly intervals for the first three months of treatment. Liver function tests should be performed monthly for the first three months of treatment.
Care should be exercised in those with allergic, renal or hepatic disease.
Effects:
General: raised temperature, periorbital oedema and other allergic responses such as painful joints, inflammation of the heart and lung.
Central nervous system: headache, vertigo, tinnitus, peripheral neuropathy, ataxia, convulsions.
Respiratory: dyspnoea, cough, fibrosing alveolitis.
Gastrointestinal: nausea, loss of appetite, stomatitis, parotitis,

pancreatitis, hepatitis, exacerbation of the colitis.
Psychological: insomnia, mental depression, hallucinations.
Urogenital: crystalluria, haematuria, proteinuria, nephrotic syndrome, low sperm count, abnormal sperm.
Blood: agranulocytosis, megaloblastic anaemia, haemolytic anaemia, leucopenia, aplastic anaemia, thrombocytopenia.
Skin: generalised skin rashes, itching, urticaria, photosensitivity.
Allergic: anaphylaxis, periorbital oedema.

CHEM NAME	TRADE NAME	FORMULATION
sulphasalazine	SALAZOPYRIN	500mg, 250mg/5ml, 3G enema
	SALAZOPYRIN EN	500mg

Maintenance 4 tablets or 40ml daily in divided doses.
Suppositories two morning and at night after defaecation.

CORTICOSTEROID

Category III drugs.
This is added to many local applications since it has anti-inflammatory and soothing effects.
Here they are of low potency and there will be less severe effects of mucosal thinning and damage. However, they will mask the real picture.

CHEM NAME	TRADE NAME	FORMULATION
betamethasone	BETNOVATE RECTAL	with phenylephrine, lignocaine (ointment)

With the addition of a sympathomimetic agent (vasoconstrictor) and a local anaesthetic.

fluocortolone	ULTRAPROCT	with cinchocaine (suppositories,ointment)

With the addition of a local anaesthetic.

hydrocortisone	ANUGESIC-HC	with pramoxine, zinc oxide, Peru balsam, benzyl benzoate, bismuth oxide (cream, suppositories)

With the addition of soothing and antiseptic agents.

	ANUSOL HC	with benzyl benzoate, bismuth subgallate,

bismuth oxide, Peru
balsam, zinc oxide
(ointment,
suppositories)

With the addition of astringents and antiseptics.

COLIFOAM   10% foam

Used for ulcerative colitis, proctitis.
1 applicatorful into the rectum once or twice daily for 2 or 3 weeks.
Every second day afterwards.

PROCTOFOAM HC   with pramoxine (foam)

Used for ulcerative colitis, proctitis, haemorrhoids.
1 applicatorful into the rectum two or three times daily. For anal
conditions apply as required.
With the addition of a local anaesthetic.

PROCTOSEDYL   5mg with cinchocaine
(ointment,suppositories)

With the addition of a local anaesthetic.

UNIROID   5mg with neomycin,
polymyxin B,
cinchocaine
(ointment,suppositories)

With the addition of antibiotics and a local anaesthetic.

XYLOPROCT   5mg with lignocaine, zinc
oxide, aluminium
acetate
(ointment,suppositories)

With the addition of local anaesthetic.

prednisolone   ANACAL   with heparinoid,
lauromacrogol 400,
hexachlorophane
(ointment,suppositories)

With the addition of soothing and antiseptic agents.

PREDENEMA   20mg enema

One nightly for two to four weeks.
For ulcerative colitis.

PREDFOAM   20mg foam

1–2 daily for 2–4 weeks.
For ulcerative colitis.

PREDSOL   20mg enema

1 at night for 2–4 weeks.
For ulcerative colitis.

SCHERIPROCT   with cinchocaine
(ointment,suppositories)

With the addition of a local anaesthetic.

COMMENTS

All of these compounds are used to relieve symptoms of discomfort, inflammation and itching. They are usually prescribed empirically depending on the particular favourite of the practitioner and the appearance of the condition. If infection is suspected then a compound containing an antibiotic will be given.

If anti-inflammatory or corticosteroid compounds are given alone in cases of infection then this will worsen.

They are suppressive in terms of energetic medicine and so removal may result in a flare-up of symptoms dependent on the severity of the condition, the duration of treatment and the dosage and frequency of applications.

Table of drugs in order of increasing strength:

CATEGORY I
- drugs taken symptomatically

CATEGORY II
- soothing agents
- antiseptic/local anaesthetics
- salicylate
- salicylate-sulphonamide

CATEGORY III
- corticosteroids — rectal
- corticosteroids — oral

10   CENTRAL NERVOUS SYSTEM

ANALGESICS

These are widely available for the treatment of pain and/or fever. Compounds containing aspirin or paracetamol have an effect on lowering temperature. Many formulations are available over-the-counter. It is helpful to directly question regarding this since there are over 100 medications available which contain aspirin for example.

The condition of analgesic nephropathy was recognised in 1953 as being due to the intake of phenacetin and resulted in its removal from the market. However this condition can be initiated by most of the analgesics in use today including the non-steroidal anti-inflammatory agents used in the treatment of arthritis. Around 3% of cases of renal failure are analgesic-induced although there are variations around the world. Spain has a very low proportion (0.3%) whilst Switzerland has a relatively high proportion (17.5%).

SALICYLATE

Category II drug.

Aspirin (salicylic acid) is the best example of this group of drugs. It is widely used for pain relief and in the treatment of arthritic disorders since there is also an anti-inflammatory effect. In cases of rheumatoid arthritis very high doses of aspirin may be used.

Aspirin is also a common component of over-the-counter remedies and it is essential to enquire about such drugs.

Aspirin should not be given to children under the age of 12 years because of Reye's syndrome — a severe illness characterised by liver and kidney damage which may be fatal.

Contraindications:

Active peptic ulcer, haemophilia.

Aspirin should not be given to children under the age of 12 years because of the risk of Reye's syndrome. This is a potentially fatal condition leading to liver and kidney damage. Reye's syndrome is mainly seen in those between 6 months and 15 years.

Precautions:

Caution in people with a history of peptic ulceration. It can induce gastrointestinal haemorrhage of a major degree.

Aspirin can precipitate wheezing in asthmatic patients and in some susceptible people.

Effects:

Central nervous system: tinnitus.

Respiratory: asthma.

Gastrointestinal: blood loss (chronic and acute) — this mainly occurs if over 15 tablets per week are taken and can be seen even in intravenous administration. Anaemia is the result in 10–15% of patients on continuous treatment with arthritis.

Nausea, vomiting, constipation, diarrhoea, indigestion.

Liver damage.

Urogenital: kidney stones, worsening of menorrhagia, increased blood loss at delivery.

There is a possible role in the development and maintenance of analgesic nephropathy.

Allergy: hypersensitivity reactions.

Blood: thrombocytopenia, aplastic anaemia, agranulocytosis, pancytopenia, haemolytic anaemia, macrocytic anaemia.

Skin: urticaria, eczema, purpura, erythema nodosum, pustular psoriasis.

Special senses: some workers have suggested a role in impairment of hearing by continued use. Certainly overdosage leads to headache, tinnitus, a sensation of pressure as if the ear were filled with water, impaired hearing and vertigo.

CHEM NAME	TRADE NAME	FORMULATION
aspirin	ASPAV	500mg with 10mg papaveretum

1 or 2 every four to six hours. Maximum of 8 in 24 hours. With the addition of an opiate.

	ANGETTES	75mg

Given to patients after a myocardial infarction to prevent a second attack or those with severe angina pectoris.
2 daily. May be given in doses of 4 daily for the treatment of unstable angina pectoris.

	ASPIRIN	300mg

300–900mg every four to six hours. Maximum 4G daily.

	CAPRIN	324mg

3 three or four times daily.

	NU–SEALS Aspirin	300mg, 600 mg – enteric coated

3 three or four times daily. Maximum 8G daily in arthritis.

	PLATET	300mg

Given to patients after a myocardial infarction to prevent a second attack or those with severe angina pectoris.1 daily.

SOLPRIN	300mg

1–3 every four to six hours. Maximum 12 daily. In cases of arthritis the maximum is 8G daily with a usual dose of 4G daily.

CO-CODAPRIN DISPERSIBLE	400mg with 8mg codeine phosphate

1–2 every four to six hours.
With the addition of an opiate.

CODIS	400mg with 8mg codeine phosphate

1–2 four hourly. Maximum 8 in 24 hours.
With the addition of an opiate.

EQUAGESIC	250mg with 75mg ethoheptazine, 150mg meprobamate

2 three or four times daily.
Controlled drug.
With the addition of an opiate and a tranquilliser.

HYPON	325mg with 10mg caffeine, 5mg codeine phosphate

1–2 four hourly.
With the addition of a xanthine and an opiate.

LABOPRIN	300mg with 245mg lysine

1–3 four hourly.

ROBAXISAL FORTE	325mg with 400mg methocarbamol

Used in the treatment of muscle spasm.
2 four times daily.
Elderly: 1 four times daily.
With the addition of a carbamate tranquilliser.

aloxiprin   PALAPRIN FORTE   600mg
Adults and children: 1 tablet per 6.5Kg body-weight daily.

choline magnesium TRILISATE   500mg
  trisalicylate
2–3 twice daily.
Not for children.

diflusinal   DOLOBID   250mg, 500mg
Maintenance 250–500mg twice daily.

salsalate   DISALCID   500mg
2 three or four times daily.
Not for children.

OPIATE

Category II.

These are derived from the opium poppy and there are several examples of differing strengths.

Heroin is noted for producing a sense of euphoria and well-being in which unpleasant symptoms such as anxiety, pain and so on seem unimportant. All the opiates have the same effect.

Withdrawal leads to symptoms which occur anytime between a few hours and 24–48 hours. The most severe go by 10 days.

They include anxiety, restlessness, insomnia, irritability, general aches and pains, yawning, runny eyes and nose, sweating, increased temperature, increased respiratory rate, raised blood pressure, abdominal cramps, dehydration, anorexia, loss of weight.

Although these may be extreme in the case of heroin withdrawal they are seen in mild forms with codeine and dihydrocodeine.

Contraindications:

Respiratory depression, obstructive airways disease, chronic lung disease, hypotension, asthma, hepatic disease, head injury, concurrent administration of MAOI or within two weeks of their use.

Precautions:

Asthma, the elderly, hypothyroidism and renal or hepatic disease.

Effects:

General: drowsiness.

Cardiovascular: hypertension.

Respiratory: respiratory depression, cough supression.

Central nervous system: headache, vertigo, analgesia.

Gastrointestinal: anorexia, nausea, vomiting, constipation.

Psychological: mood changes, mental impairment.

Urogenital: urinary retention, oliguria.

Skin: itching, urticaria, sweating.

CHEM NAME	TRADE NAME	FORMULATION
buprenorphine	TEMGESIC	0.2mg
1–2 six to eight hourly or as required.		
Controlled drug.		
codeine phosphate	CODEINE PHOSPHATE	15mg, 30mg, 60mg
10–60mg every four hours as required. Maximum 200mg daily.		
dextromoramide	PALFIUM	5mg, 10mg, 10mg

suppository
Suppository: 1 as required.
Tablets: up to 5mg initially then adjusted according to response.
Controlled drug.

| dextro- | DOLOXENE | 60mg |
| propoxyphene | | |

1 three or four times daily.

	CO-PROXAMOL	32.5mg with 325mg paracetamol
	DISTALGESIC	32.5mg with 325mg paracetamol
	PAXALGESIC	32.5mg with 325mg paracetamol

2 three or four times daily.
With the addition of a paracetamol analgesic.

| | DOLOXENE CO | 65mg with 375mg aspirin, 30mg caffeine |

1 three or four times daily.
With the addition of a salicylate analgesic and a xanthine.
This drug can produce respiratory depression easily and even apnoea.
For this reason it is implicated in overdose deaths even at relatively
low levels particularly if taken with other central nervous system
depressants such as alcohol or tranquillisers.
It is also associated with the development of euphoria and even
hallucinations.

| dihydrocodeine | CO-DYDRAMOL | 10mg with 500mg paracetamol |

1–2 tablets every four to six hours when necessary. Maximum 8 daily.
ith the addition of a paracetamol analgesic.

| | DF118 | 30mg, 10mg/5ml |

1 tablet or 5–15ml four to six hourly.

| | DHC CONTINUS | 60mg sustained-release 1 every twelve hours. |

| dipipanone | DICONAL | 10mg with 30mg cyclizine |

Maximum 1 initially.
Controlled drug.
With the addition of an antiemetic.

| methadone | PHYSEPTONE | 5mg |

5–10mg six to eight hourly.
Controlled drug.
This may cause the development of involuntary choreiform
movements of the upper body and arms.

| morphine | MST CONTINUS | 10mg, 30mg, 60mg, 100mg |

10–20mg twice daily then adjusted according to response.
Controlled drug.

phenazocine   NARPHEN   5mg
1 four to six hourly. Maximum single dose 20mg.

OPIATE AGONIST-ANTAGONIST

Category II drug.
This is a general group with diverse mechanisms of action.

MEPTAZINOL

Precautions:
Hepatic or renal insufficiency, respiratory depression, head injuries, myocardial infarction.
Effects:
General: left sided chest pain.
Central nervous system: dizziness, vertigo, headache.
Psychological: sleepiness.
Gastrointestinal: anorexia, nausea, vomiting, constipation, diarrhoea, abdominal pain, dyspepsia.
Special senses: tinnitus.
Skin: increased sweating, rash.

CHEM NAME	TRADE NAME	FORMULATION
meptazinol	MEPTID	200mg

1 three to six hourly as required.

NEFOPAM

Category II.
Contraindications:
History of convulsions, myocardial infarction and those taking MAOI.
Precautions:
Hepatic or renal insufficiency, concurrent use of tricyclic anti-depressants, anticholinergics or sympathomimetics and if a risk of urinary retention.
Effects:
General: lightheadedness.
Cardiovascular: rapid pulse, palpitations.
Central nervous system: headache.

Psychological: nervousness, insomnia.
Gastrointestinal: nausea, vomiting, dry mouth.
Urogenital: pink discolouration of the urine.
Skin: sweating.
Special senses: blurred vision.

CHEM NAME	TRADE NAME	FORMULATION
nefopam	ACUPAN	30mg

1–3 three times daily.

PENTAZOCINE

Category II.
Contraindications:
Respiratory depression, raised intracranial pressure, head injuries and pathological brain conditions where clouding of consciousness may occur.
Precautions:
Impaired renal or hepatic function.
Effects:
General: sedation.
Respiratory: respiratory depression.
Central nervous system: vertigo.
Psychological: hallucinations (more than with the opiates), dysphoria.
Gastrointestinal: nausea, vomiting.
Skin: increased sweating, skin flushes.
Special senses: visual disturbances.
Withdrawal symptoms are mild abdominal cramps, nausea, vomiting, nervousness, irritability, insomnia, restlessness, dizziness, fever and chills. This has mainly been reported after long-term usage of injectable forms.

CHEM NAME	TRADE NAME	FORMULATION
pentazocine	FORTAGESIC	15mg with 500mg paracetamol

2 up to four times daily.
Children: under 7 years not recommended, 7–12 years 1 every three to four hours to a maximum of 4 doses daily.
With the addition of a paracetamol analgesic.

	FORTRAL	25mg, 50mg

25–100mg three to four hourly after meals.

Children: under 1 year not recommended, 1–6 years injection only,
6–12 years 25mg three to four hourly.
Controlled drug.

PARACETAMOL ANALGESIC

Category II drug.
A very commonly taken analgesic. On a par with aspirin in
terms of effectiveness and severity. It is used much more in
children now since aspirin has been banned for this age group.
The main problem is with liver damage when excessive doses
are taken. This is usually seen in overdose where more than 10G
can lead to problems. However overuse has caused damage in
some people when taken for prolonged fever or pain.
Precautions:
Sodium is often contained in the tablets and this should be
taken into account when given to patients with cardiac failure,
oedema or hypertension for whom excess sodium intake may
be harmful. It may worsen the wheezing in those who are
sensitive to aspirin.
Effects:
There are toxic effects on the liver when taken as a large single
dose. Hepatic failure may result unless antidoted within about
48 hours. This is a significant cause of death from drug
overdosage. Renal damage and pancreatitis may also result.
Alcoholics, those receiving barbiturates and those who are
chronically malnourished are more sensitive to these toxic
effects.
Long term use may lead to renal damage and ultimately renal
failure.
Analgesic nephropathy is a well-described condition 9 and
even occurs where doses have been within 'safe' limits.
Blood: thrombocytopenia, agranulocytosis.

CHEM NAME	TRADE NAME	FORMULATION
paracetamol	CALPOL INFANT	120mg/5ml
	DISPROL PAED.	120mg/5ml
	PALDESIC	120mg/5ml
	PANALEVE	120mg/5ml
	SALZONE	120mg/5ml

Under 3 months not recommended, 3–12 months 2.5–5ml, 1–6 years
5–10ml.
Both four times daily.

CAFADOL   500mg with 30mg caffeine

2 three to four hourly.
Children: under 5 years not recommended, 5–12 years half adult dose.
With the addition of a xanthine.

CALPOL SIX PLUS   250mg/5ml

Adults: 10–20ml four times daily.
Children: 6–12 years 5–10ml four times daily.

CO-CODAMOL   500mg with 8mg codeine
                                           phosphate

1–2 every 4–6 hours. Maximum 8 daily.
With the addition of an opiate.

FORMULIX   120mg/5ml with 12mg
                                           codeine phosphate

Children: under 3 years not recommended, 3–6 years 5ml, 7–12 years
10ml. Both three or four times daily.
With the addition of an opiate.

LOBAK   450mg with 100mg
                                           chlormezanone

Used in the treatment of muscle spasm.
1–2 three times daily. Not more than 8 in 24 hours.
Elderly: half dose.
Not for children.
With the addition of a tranquilliser.

MEDISED   120mg with 2.5mg
                                           promethazine/5ml

Under 3 months not recommended, 3–12 months 5ml, 1–6 years 10ml,
6–12 years 20ml. All up to maximum of four times daily.
With the addition of an antihistamine.

MEDISED TABLETS   500mg with 10mg
                                           promethazine.

Two at night or at four hourly intervals. Maximum of 8 daily.
Children: not recommended.
With the addition of an antihistamine.

PAMETON   500mg with 250mg
                                           methionine

2 tablets up to four times daily.
Children: under 6 years not recommended, 6–12 years half–1 tablet
four hourly. Maximum 4 doses daily.
With the addition of a paracetamol antidote.
NOTE.
This is included in some formulations of paracetamol so that if
overdosage does occur there is a ready-made supply of antidote
already ingested.
It is a reflection of the powerful effect of paracetamol.

PANADOL   500mg

2 three or four times daily.

Children: under 6 years not recommended, 6–12 years half–1 every 4 hours. Maximum 4 doses daily.

PARACODOL	500mg with 8mg codeine phosphate

1–2 four to six hourly. Maximum 8 in 24 hours.
Children: under 6 years not recommended, 6–12 years half–1.
Maximum 4 doses daily.
With the addition of an opiate.

PARAHYPON	500mg with 10mg caffeine, 5mg codeine phosphate

1–2 four times daily.
Children: under 6 years not recommended, 6–12 years half adult dose.
With the addition of a xanthine and an opiate.

PARAKE	500mg with 8mg codeine phosphate

2 four hourly. Maximum 8 in 24 hours.
Not for children.
With the addition of an opiate.

PARAMOL	500mg with 10mg dihydrocodeine

1 four hourly increasing to 2 four times daily if necessary.
Not for children.
With the addition of an opiate.

PARDALE	400mg with 9mg codeine phosphate, 10mg caffeine

1–2 three or four times daily.
Not for children.
With the addition of an opiate and a xanthine.

PROPAIN	400mg with 10mg codeine phosphate, 5mg diphenhydramine, 50mg caffeine

1–2 four hourly. Maximum 10 daily.
Not for children.
With the addition of an opiate, an antihistamine and a xanthine.

SOLPADOL	500mg with 30mg codeine phosphate

2 every four hours. Not more than 6 in 24 hours.
Not for children.
With the addition of an opiate.

SYNDOL	450mg with 10mg codeine phosphate, 5mg doxylamine, 30mg

	caffeine

1–2 four to six hourly. Maximum 8 daily.
Not for children.
With the addition of an opiate, an antihistamine and a xanthine.

TYLEX	500mg with 30mg codeine phosphate

1–2 every four hours. Maximum 6 daily.
Not for children.
With the addition of an opiate.

COMMENTS

There are many different types of analgesic used but the main ones are salicylates (aspirin), paracetamol and opiates (morphine and its derivatives). When taken occasionally for the relief of pain there will be minimal harmful effects but they are often used regularly, daily and in significant doses.

Phenacetin used regularly caused renal damage and so was removed from the market but any analgesic used in this way can harm renal function. This is particularly true in the elderly and in those conditions where chronic pain is a feature. It is commonly the case that the kidneys may already be involved in the disease process, e.g. rheumatoid arthritis[10].

As a group there are many similarities between the analgesics and non-steroidal anti-inflammatory drugs. There are similar effects and side-effects particularly in the case of aspirin.

Opiates have mental effects as well as relieving pain and these can lead to sedation, drowsiness, confusion in the elderly and withdrawal symptoms of anxiety, restlessness and insomnia. All opiates have this ability although there are differing strengths.

The following opiates are listed in order of severity:

CATEGORY II
- codeine phosphate
- dextroproxyphene
- dihydrocodeine
- methadone
- dextromoramide, dipipanone, levorphanol, morphine, phenazocine

Symptomatic use of any analgesic would place it in Category I.

The other analgesics, aspirin and paracetamol being the main examples, affect other areas. Aspirin has a predilection for the gastrointestinal tract so indigestion, peptic ulceration and upper gastrointestinal haemorrhage occur.

Paracetamol in large doses damages the liver and overdosage can cause fatal hepatic necrosis.

Both drugs, used regularly, can cause renal damage and my feeling is that analgesics are a major cause of debility, ill-health and kidney-related disease in the elderly. Low backache, frequency and nocturia are common.

Treatment needs to be directed at the painful condition whilst reducing the analgesics perhaps with the prescription of less powerful agents.

Although analgesics relieve pain they do so to a variable degree. Musculoskeletal problems are particularly resistant. In the long term of course they may lead to more pain because of their depleting effect.

Migraine

Betablockers are also used in the treatment of migraine to prevent attacks and so they are taken regularly. They are listed on page 99 rather than repeated here. The same approach should be taken with them whatever their indication.

Migraine as understood by conventional sources is in fact a mixed bag of conditions with varying clinical pictures. There may be upper gastrointestinal symptoms such as nausea and vomiting, there may be a large psychological component, there may be precipitation by foods. They are all considered as a single entity by conventional medicine and the same drugs are used in most cases.

The ergotamines are less commonly used now due to their severe side-effects.

ERGOTAMINE

Category II.

Withdrawal of this drug after chronic use may lead to the appearance of headaches. This may result in further administration of the drug. The total dose required to lead to this may be as small as 10mg per week. This level leads to effects such as those listed below in half of patients.

Contraindications:
Atherosclerosis, coronary artery disease, thrombophlebitis, Raynaud's syndrome, Buerger's disease and where there is liver or kidney dysfunction.

Effects:
Cardiovascular: ECG changes and angina pectoris in those susceptible, leg cramps, postural hypotension, fainting.
The danger with this drug is that constriction of blood vessels occur leading to coldness and pallor of the extremities and in severe cases (usually with large doses) gangrene.
Central nervous system: vertigo, increased headache.
Gastrointestinal: nausea, vomiting, abdominal pain, diarrhoea.

CHEM NAME	TRADE NAME	FORMULATION
ergotamine	LINGRAINE	2mg

1 at onset of attack, repeated if necessary 30–60 minutes later. Maximum 3 in 24 hours, 6 in any one week.

	MEDIHALER-ERGOTAMINE	inhaler (0.36mg/dose)

1 dose repeated if required after five minutes. Maximum 6 doses in 24 hours, 15 in any one week.

	CAFERGOT	1mg with 100mg caffeine

1 or 2 at onset of attack. Maximum 4 daily, 10 in any one week.
With the addition of a xanthine.

	CAFERGOT SUPPOSITORIES	2mg with 100mg caffeine

1 at onset of attack. Maximum 2 daily, 5 in any one week.
With the addition of a xanthine.

	MIGRIL	2mg with 50mg cyclizine 100mg caffeine

1–2 at onset of attack then half–1 at half hourly intervals. Maximum 4 per attack, 6 in any one week.
With the addition of an antihistamine and a xanthine.

SEROTONIN ANTAGONIST

These are used in the belief that it is abnormalities of chemical balance which is responsible for migraine.

METHYSERGIDE

Category II.
    This drug is to be taken regularly each day to prevent attacks

of migraine. It is related to LSD (lysergic acid diethylamide).
Contraindications:
Peripheral vascular disorders, progressive arteriosclerosis, severe hypertension, coronary heart disease, phlebitis or cellulitis of the lower extremities, pulmonary disease, collagen disease, impaired liver or kidney function, diseases of the urinary tract, cachectic or septic conditions, psychological disorders.
Precautions:
Continuous administration should not exceed 6 months without at least one month for reassessment. Dosage must be reduced gradually over two or three weeks to reduce the risk of rebound headaches.
Regular clinical supervision is essential.
Attention should be paid to symptoms of urinary dysfunction, pain in the loin, flank or chest and pain, coldness or numbness in the limbs.
Patients should be regularly examined for vascular, cardiac or abdominal signs.
Care is needed if there is a past history of peptic ulceration.
Effects:
General: tiredness, drowsiness.
Cardiovascular: oedema, leg cramps, rapid heart rate, postural hypotension, angina pectoris, heart murmurs due to heart valve fibrosis which may lead to heart failure in some.
Vascular spasm may be induced leading to coldness, numbness and pain in the limbs, hypertension, angina pectoris and reversible loss of vision depending on the vessel involved.
Central nervous system: dizziness.
Psychological: insomnia, mental and behavioural disturbances, restlessness, LSD-like reaction.
Gastrointestinal: nausea, heartburn, abdominal discomfort.
Skin: rashes, loss of head hair.
Retroperitoneal fibrosis is a risk with continuous treatment although this is minimised by having a break from medication for at least one month every six. This condition leads to constriction of arteries, veins and lymphatic vessels which may cause bowel damage.
Fibrosis in other areas such as pericardium, heart, blood vessels and lungs may also occur.
Blood: haemolytic anaemia, neutropenia, eosinophilia.

CHEM NAME	TRADE NAME	FORMULATION
methysergide	DESERIL	1mg

1–2 two or three times daily.

PIZOTIFEN

Category II drug.
This is taken regularly each day to prevent attacks.
Precautions:
Glaucoma (closed-angle), predisposition to urinary retention and renal insufficiency.
Effects:
General: drowsiness.
Central nervous system: dizziness.
Gastrointestinal: nausea, weight gain, increased appetite.

CHEM NAME	TRADE NAME	FORMULATION
pizotifen	SANOMIGRAN	0.5mg, 1.5mg, 0.25mg/5ml

Usually 1.5mg daily. Maximum 6mg daily.

SYMPATHOMIMETIC AGENT

Category II drug.
These are used in asthma as well as cough remedies where they are described in more detail (see page 167).

CHEM NAME	TRADE NAME	FORMULATION
isometheptene	MIDRID	65mg with 325mg paracetamol

2 at once then 1 every hour. Maximum 5 in 12 hours.
With the addition of a paracetamol analgesic.

ANTIDOPAMINERGIC AGENT

Category II drug.
Widely used as an antiemetic. See page 181 for more details.

CHEM NAME	TRADE NAME	FORMULATION
metoclopramide	MIGRAVESS	5mg with 325mg aspirin
	MIGRAVESS FORTE	5mg with 450mg aspirin

2 at onset of attack, maximum 6 daily.
With the addition of a salicylate analgesic.

	TRADE NAME	FORMULATION
	PARAMAX	5mg with 500mg paracetamol

Over 20 years, 2 at onset of attack, then 2 four hourly with a maximum of 6 in 24 hours.
With the addition of a paracetamol analgesic.

PARACETAMOL ANALGESIC

Category II drug.
See analgesics on page 210 for details.

CHEM NAME	TRADE NAME	FORMULATION
paracetamol	MIGRALEVE	(pink) 500mg with 8mg codeine phosphate 6.25mg buclizine

With the addition of an opiate and an antihistamine.

		FORMULATION
		(yellow) 500mg with 8mg codeine phosphate

With the addition of an opiate.
2 pink at onset. If pain persists then 2 yellow every 4 hours. Maximum
2 pink and 6 yellow in 24

CENTRAL ALPHA AGONIST

Category III drug.
This is the same chemical as included in CATAPRES for the treatment of hypertension although in that case the dosage is higher. If taken with hypotensive agents then there may be an additive effect in lowering the blood pressure.
It is designed to prevent attacks and so is taken regularly each day. It is also prescribed to control menopausal symptoms especially where there is flushing.

Precautions:
Depression or a history of depression.
Effects:
General: sedation
Central nervous system: dizziness.
Psychological: nocturnal unrest.
Gastrointestinal: dry mouth, nausea, nocturnal unrest.
Skin: rash.

CHEM NAME	TRADE NAME	FORMULATION
clonidine 2–3 twice daily.	DIXARIT	25mcg

COMMENTS

Energetically migraine is a mixed bag of conditions. However, in conventional medicine all of these are considered together and treatments are very much the same in different cases.
Drugs may be taken for an attack — MIGRALEVE, LINGRAINE, CAFERGOT, MIGRIL, MIDRID, MIGRAVESS and PARAMAX — when they may relieve the headache and associated symptoms such as vomiting. They are of variable effectiveness and many people find that rest is a major factor which affects an acute attack.
Prophylaxis with agents such as DIXARIT, DESERIL, SANOMIGRAN and betablockers is initiated if attacks are frequent and severe. They definitely stop or ameliorate the severity and frequency of attacks but, of course, lead to other problems either as side-effects or perhaps a change in the site of the pathology.
Treatment in these cases is more difficult because the drugs hide the clinical picture. It may be necessary, in order to make a correct diagnosis, to reduce the tablets slightly until symptoms appear.

Parkinson's Disease

Parkinson's disease is a disease of the central nervous system characterised by tremor, rigidity and slowness of movement. It is due to imbalances in the basal ganglia which make up part of the extrapyramidal system. This serves to exercise some control over the voluntary motor system.

The imbalance is seen as being chemical by Western medicine. Therefore, chemicals are given to try and restore the 'normal' state of affairs. Dopamine is in short supply in the Parkinsonian patient and so this is added (or drugs with similar actions) or drugs are given which destroy the chemicals having the opposite effect as dopamine (anticholinergic agents).

The usual cause is atherosclerotic degeneration although drugs, particularly the antipsychotic agents. can be implicated. Antidopaminergic drugs (see nausea and vomiting — see page 181) may also cause Parkinsonian symptoms.

DOPAMINERGIC

Category II drug.

This has similar actions on the brain as dopamine. It is also used in certain viral diseases due to its antiviral effect (see page 51).

Contraindications:

History of gastric ulceration, those subject to convulsions and severe renal disease.

Precautions:

Confusional or hallucinatory states, renal impairment, liver disease and congestive cardiac failure.

The use of this drug with other anti-Parkinsonian agents may lead to increased effects of these other drugs.

Effects:

General: lethargy.

Cardiovascular: peripheral oedema.

Gastrointestinal: nausea, dry mouth.

Central nervous system: dizziness, convulsions.

Psychological: nervousness, insomnia, feeling of detachment, psychotic symptoms of mania, hallucinations, agitation and confusion (more likely when dosage 200mg per day or more).

Skin: rashes.

Special senses: blurred vision.

CHEM NAME	TRADE NAME	FORMULATION
amantadine	MANTADINE	100mg
	SYMMETREL	100mg, 50mg/5ml
100mg twice daily.		

ANTICHOLINERGIC

Category II drug.
These are also used in asthma, diarrhoea and upper abdominal conditions — see page 173 for full details.

CHEM NAME	TRADE NAME	FORMULATION
benzhexol	ARTANE	2mg,5mg
	BENTEX	2mg, 5mg
	BROFLEX	5mg/5ml

Maintenance, usually 5–15mg daily. Maximum 20mg daily.
This drug is especially likely to produce excitement and acute confusional states even at fairly low doses.

benztropine	COGENTIN	2mg

As required to maximum 6mg daily.
This drug especially produces sedation. Patients must be warned definitely not to drive. Other effects include rashes, peripheral numbness and muscular weakness.

methixene	TREMONIL	5mg

3–12 daily.
Elderly, usual maintenance 3–6 daily.

orphenadine	BIORPHEN	25mg/5ml
	DISIPAL	50mg

Maintenance, usually 100–300mg daily. Maximum 400mg daily.

procyclidine	ARPICOLIN	2.5mg, 5mg/5ml
	KEMADRIN	5mg

Usual maximum 30mg daily.

DOPAMINE AGONIST

Category II drug.
This has similar actions on the brain as dopamine.
This drug is used for several conditions such as endocrine disease due to oversecretion of prolactin, e.g. infertility, some pituitary tumours, Parkinson's disease, cyclical breast disorders such as PMS.
Precautions:
Gynaecological assessment including cervical smear and D and C should be performed on women taking this drug for long periods. This should be done six-monthly for post-menopausal and annually for pre-menopausal women.

Severe cardiovascular disease or those with a history of psychotic illness.

Pleural effusions may develop in elderly patients on high dose, long-term treatment and so breathlessness and cough should be checked.

Fibrosis in the retroperitoneal tissues may also occur (with doses over 30mg for more than a year) and so back pain, kidney symptoms and oedema of the lower limbs should be asked about and investigated.

Effects:

General: drowsiness..

Cardiovascular: slow pulse rate (may manifest as palpitations), hypotension, worsening of angina pectoris, leg cramps, attacks of reversible pallor of the fingers and toes induced by the cold.

Central nervous system: dizziness, headache, migraine (this may be precipitated by alcohol), dyskinesia in those being treated for Parkinson's disease, fainting, parasthesiae.

Psychological: confusion, agitation and excitation, hallucinations, delusions, paranoia, bad dreams.

Gastrointestinal: nausea, vomiting, constipation, liver function changes.

Skin: flushing.

Special senses: nasal catarrh, blurred vision, double vision.

Blood: leucocytopenia, thrombocytopenia.

CHEM NAME	TRADE NAME	FORMULATION
bromocryptine	PARLODEL	1mg, 2.5mg
30–75mg daily in Parkinson's disease.		
2.5–5.0mg daily in prostatic tumours and to suppress lactation.		
lysuride	REVANIL	200mcg
Gradual increase in dose as required to maximum of 25 tablets daily.		

DOPAMINE PRECURSOR

Category II drug.

The definitive answer in conventional medicine since it is lack of dopamine which is seen as the main issue. However early use of this drug may result in long-term deterioration. In addition there is the appearance of the 'on-off' effect after chronic use. The patient swings between periods of normal mobility with severe adverse drug effects and periods of severe parkinsonian symptoms with no adverse drug effects.

Contraindications:
Narrow-angle glaucoma, severe psychoneuroses or psychoses, with MAOI or within 2 weeks of their withdrawal and if there is malignant melanoma or a history of this.

Precautions:
Vitamin B6 will block the effects of this drug.

Caution with endocrine, renal, hepatic, pulmonary disease, cardiovascular disease especially where there is a history of myocardial infarction, peptic ulceration, where sympathomimetic drugs may be used, e.g. bronchial asthma, and with antihypertensive drugs.

Regular tests of liver function, blood count, renal and cardiovascular function should be performed.

Effects:
General: weakness, gout.

Cardiovascular: hypotension — usually when rising or standing, ventricular arrhythmias in those with cardiac disease, hypertension.

Central nervous system: headache, peripheral neuropathy.

Involuntary movements usually in the form of oral dyskinesia but which may also affect the tongue, lips, jaw or trunk It may continue for days or months after the drug has been stopped.

There may be sudden attacks of heaviness in the feet and an inability to begin walking. There is an associated trembling of the legs and the patient often falls forward.

Psychological: mild elation, depression (1 in 10), anxiety, agitation, aggression, hallucinations and delusions, confusion (1 in 8), sleep disturbances (1 in 5).

Gastrointestinal: nausea, vomiting, anorexia (these three symptoms occur in 30–80% of patients initially), liver function test changes.

Urogenital: reddish discolouration of urine — not blood, urinary retention.

Skin: flushing.

Blood: leucopenia, fall in haemoglobin levels, thrombocytopenia.

CHEM NAME	TRADE NAME	FORMULATION
levodopa	BROCADOPA	125mg, 250mg, 550mg
	LARODOPA	500mg
Usually 1–8G daily.		
	MADOPAR '62.5'	50mg with 12.5mg benserazide

MADOPAR '125'	100mg with 25mg benserazide
MADOPAR '250'	200mg with 50mg benserazide
MADOPAR CR	100mg with 25mg benserazide continuous release

Usual maintenance 4–8 x '125' daily in divided doses.
Elderly, initially 1 x '62.6' once or twice daily increasing by 1 x '62.5' as required.
With the addition of a decarboxylase inhibitor.

SINEMET 'LS'	50mg with 12.5mg carbidopa
SINEMET '110'	100mg with 10mg carbidopa
SINEMET 'PLUS'	100mg with 25mg carbidopa
SINEMET '275'	250mg with 25mg carbidopa

Equivalent of 6x'PLUS' daily.
With the addition of a decarboxylase inhibitor.
NOTE
Carbidopa (a decarboxylase inhibitor) is combined with a dopamine precursor (levodopa) so that a lower dose of the latter is needed.
This is reputed to reduce side-effects.

MONOAMINE OXIDASE-B INHIBITOR

Category II drug.
This drug must be viewed as the monoamine oxidase inhibitors used in the treatment of depression. Therefore similar comments are applicable here. See page 68 for full details of those.
Precautions:
This drug may increase the side-effects of levodopa leading to the appearance of involuntary movements and/or agitation.
Effects:
Cardiovascular: low blood pressure.
Psychological: confusion, psychosis.
Gastrointestinal: nausea.

CHEM NAME	TRADE NAME	FORMULATION
selegiline	ELDEPRYL	5mg

2 daily.
This drug is often used in conjunction with levodopa treatment.

COMMENTS

Parkinson's disease is a chronic degenerative disorder of the central nervous system characterised by tremor, rigidity and slowness of movement.

Drug treatment only helps relieve some of the worst symptoms in the short-term — there is no claim to cure — and side-effects are common. It is clear from the lists of effects that most of these drugs are 'hot' in nature and stimulating in their action.

There may be several clinical appearances when Parkinson's disease is treated by drugs. Patients with a marked degree of rigidity tend to become more mobile but develop an increase in tremor — those with a marked degree of tremor tend to shake less but develop an increase in rigidity.

With long-term treatment there may come a point where the drugs seem to be ineffective and only produce adverse effects with anxiety, slow or no movement and unsteadiness. Here the drugs may be given intermittently to regain some effectiveness. There is increasing evidence that drugs may lead to acceleration of the degenerative process if used too early.[11]

Therefore, the primary effect is symptomatic. Alternative treatment may benefit but it is important to be aware that drug withdrawal leads to exacerbation of the tremor, rigidity and slow movement depending upon the individual case. If patients are treated early enough then response can be very good. In chronic cases with long term use of drugs then it is more difficult to obtain improvement.

Parkinson's disease can be a very rewarding condition to treat. Reduction of drug dosage removes many of the side-effects especially those of anxiety and insomnia. Treatment at the same time can definitely strengthen people so their original symptoms improve.

Epilepsy

There are several different types of epilepsy. It is diagnosed by the clinical history and the EEG appearance.

The drugs below are used in each particular type as indicated. There are general comments which can be applied to the anticonvulsants as a group. You should consider them all to belong to Category III.

Precautions:
There is a two to threefold increase in the number of foetal abnormalities when these drugs are used in pregnancy and patients should be told that there is a 90% chance of a normal child. If pregnancy does occur when they are taken then investigation for foetal abnormality is undertaken.

Periodic tests must be performed of serum calcium, alkaline phosphatase and phosphate when long term treatment is given. There may be the appearance of rickets in children and osteomalacia in adults particularly in those who are institutionalised. Regular monitoring of these levels is especially important in such patients.

Effects:
Central nervous system: ataxia, dyskinesia.
Psychological: impairment of intellectual function and memory, psychotic syndromes.
Endocrine: hypothyroidism.

CARBONIC ANHYDRASE INHIBITOR

Category III drug when used for epilepsy. Category II for its other indications.

This drug is used as drops for glaucoma and as tablets for glaucoma, epilepsy, oedema and some cases of Meniere's disease.

It is mostly used for petit mal epilepsy in children although has some effect on other types in adults.

Contraindications:
Addison's disease or any type of adrenal gland failure, renal insuffiency, precoma due to hepatic cirrhosis and hypersensitivity to sulphonamides.

Precautions:
Increasing the dose does not increase the diuretic effect but may increase the incidence of drowsiness and/or parasthesia. Also, fatigue, excitement, gastrointestinal upsets and increased frequency of urination have been seen. Confusion has occurred in some patients with oedema due to hepatic cirrhosis and these should be closely supervised.

If this drug is used for long-term treatment then patients should be specifically warned to report any unusual skin rash and periodic blood cell counts should be performed. Impairment of hearing calls for immediate cessation of the drug.

Caution in cases of prostatic hypertrophy, the elderly, those with liver dysfunction and those liable to disturbances of salt or water metabolism.

Effects:

General: fatigue, drowsiness, fever.

Respiratory: increased rate of breathing.

Central nervous system: headache, dizziness, parasthesiae of the extremities, ataxia.

Psychological: irritability, excitement, disorientation, depression.

Gastrointestinal: anorexia, vomiting, thirst, excessive drinking.

Urogenital: excessive urination, renal stones, renal disease, renal or ureteric colic, crystals in the urine, loss of libido, impotence.

Blood disorders: agranulocytosis, thrombocytopenia, leucopenia, aplastic anaemia.

Skin: flushing.

Special senses: transient myopia.

CHEM NAME	TRADE NAME	FORMULATION
acetazolamide	DIAMOX	250mg

250mg–1G daily.
Children: under 2 years 125mg daily, 2–12 years 125–750mg daily.

IMINOSTILBENE

Category III drug when used in epilepsy, Category II drug for its other indications.

This drug is used in the treatment of epilepsy and trigeminal neuralgia. It may also be used for other neuralgic pains.

Usually used for grand mal epilepsy in adults.

Contraindications:

Those taking MAOI currently or within the past two weeks.

Precautions:

The effectiveness of the oral contraceptive pill may be reduced. The blood count should be checked at regular intervals during the early stages of treatment.

Effects:

General: drowsiness.

Cardiovascular: oedema, congestive heart failure.

Respiratory: breathlessness.

Central nervous system: dizziness, peripheral neuropathy, dystonia, tremor, dyskinesia of face, mouth and tongue.

Gastrointestinal: dry mouth, diarrhoea, nausea, vomiting, jaundice, hepatitis (fatalities have occurred).
Urogenital: acute renal failure.
Blood disorders: leucopenia, thrombocytopenia, agranulocytosis, aplastic anaemia.
Skin: generalised erythematous rash in 3%.
Special senses: double vision.
A patient I treated with trigeminal neuralgia was taking this drug for relief of her pain. There was only slight amelioration of her symptoms with the drug but whenever she took it her legs became so weak that she had to use a wheelchair. Her legs were just not strong enough to support her. Whenever the drug was stopped they recovered.
It would seem that as the main action of the drug is on the central nervous system side-effects would appear in this area. With this case it was clearly due to the carbamazepine.

CHEM NAME	TRADE NAME	FORMULATION
carbamazepine	TEGRETOL	100mg, 200mg, 400mg, 100mg/5ml
	TEGRETROL RETARD	200mg, 400mg continuous-release

Usually 800mg–1.2G daily. Maximum 1.6G daily.
Children, up to 1 year, 100–200mg, 1–5 years, 200–400mg, 5–10 years, 400–600mg, 10–15 years 600–1G. All daily.

BENZODIAZEPINE

Category III drug when used for epilepsy.
See page 78 for full details of this group of drugs. In the case of epilepsy they may either be used in the acute phase to stop the convulsion or those below for prevention of attacks.

CHEM NAME	TRADE NAME	FORMULATION
clobazepam	FRISIUM	10mg

20–30mg daily. Maximum 60mg daily.
Children: under 3 years not recommended, 3–12 years, up to half adult dose.

clonazepam	RIVOTRIL	0.5mg, 2mg

Maintenance dose usually 4–8mg daily.
Elderly, initially a maximum of 0.5mg daily.
Children: up to 1 year, maintenance 0.5–1mg daily, 1–5 years

maintenance 1–3mg daily, 5–12 years maintenance 3–6mg daily.

SUCCINIMIDE

Category III drug.
Used in the treatment of petit mal epilepsy.
Effects:
General: drowsiness.
Central nervous system: ataxia, headache, dizziness, increase in number of petit mal attacks.
Psychological: apathy, drowsiness, depression, mild euphoria, psychotic states (precipitated or exacerbated).
Gastrointestinal: anorexia, gastric upset, nausea, vomiting.
Skin: rashes.
Blood disorders: leucopenia, agranulocytosis, aplastic anaemia, monocytosis, leucocytosis, eosinophilia, granulocytopenia, thrombocytopenia.
Systemic lupus erythematosus, scleroderma.

CHEM NAME	TRADE NAME	FORMULATION
ethosuximide	EMESIDE	250mg, 250mg/5ml
	ZARONTIN	250mg, 250mg/5ml

500mg daily increasing as necessary to maximum of 2G daily.
Children: under 6 years 250mg daily to maximum of 1G daily, 6–12 years as adult.

BARBITURATE

Category III drug.
Barbiturates are not used as frequently now and are mainly prescribed in cases of epilepsy. There are some patients who are still taking them for insomnia — this practice has largely stopped because of the great risk of addiction.
See page 81 for fuller details.

CHEM NAME	TRADE NAME	FORMULATION
methyl-phenobarbitone	PROMINAL	30mg, 60mg, 200mg

100–600mg daily.
Children: 5–15mg/Kg daily.
Controlled drug.

HYDANTOIN

Category III drug.
Used for grand mal and temporal lobe epilepsy. May also be given in some cases of migraine, trigeminal neuralgia and certain psychoses.

Precautions:
Liver dysfunction. There is a decreased effectiveness of the oral contraceptive when taken at the same time and the chance of pregnancy is increased 25 times as a result.

Effects:
There may be an allergic reaction of fever, breathlessness and vascular damage which is fatal in some.

General: polyarthropathy, lymphadenopathy.
Central nervous system: unsteadiness, transient hemiparesis, spasticity.
Psychological: nervousness, insomnia, hyperactivity in younger patients.
Gastrointestinal: gum overgrowth, indigestion, nausea, weight loss.
Acute liver disease developing during drug treatment is characterised by fever, rash, jaundice, enlargement of liver, spleen and lymph glands, sore throat, malaise, chills, muscle pains, generalised itching. This condition has caused deaths.
Endocrine: hyperglycaemia.
Urogenital: nephritis.
Skin: rashes, growth of hair.
Blood disorders: haemolytic anaemia, red cell aplasia, megaloblastic anaemia (well known development), leucopenia, agranulocytosis, thrombocytopenia, pancytopenia, aplastic anaemia, haemophilia (one patient developed an inhibitor to Factor 8). Scleroderma-type illness. Malignant lymphoma (very rare).

CHEM NAME	TRADE NAME	FORMULATION
phenytoin sodium	EPANUTIN	25mg, 50mg, 100mg, 30mg/5ml

100mg two to four times daily. Maximum 600mg daily.
Children: under 3 years up to 50mg three times daily, 4–6, 5–10mg/Kg, 7–12 years as adult.

PYRIMIDINEDIONE

Category III drug.
Used in grand mal and temporal lobe epilepsy.
Precautions:
Children, the elderly, debilitated patients and those with impaired function of renal, hepatic or respiratory function.
Primidone is a central nervous system depressant which is partly metabolised to phenobarbitone (see barbiturates) and so dependence may occur and a withdrawal syndrome when the drug is reduced in dosage.
Low folic acid levels are associated with long-term anticonvulsant therapy and may lead to an anaemia of the folic acid deficiency type.
Effects:
General: drowsiness, listlessness, lymphadenopathy.
Cardiovascular: oedema.
Central nervous system: headache, ataxia.
Psychological: personality changes, psychotic reactions.
Gastrointestinal: nausea, vomiting.
Endocrine: diabetes insipidus-like syndrome, thyroid gland enlargement.
Urogenital: crystalluria.
Blood: megaloblastic anaemia, other blood dyscrasias.
Skin: rashes.
Special senses: visual disturbances.
Systemic lupus erythematosus.

CHEM NAME	TRADE NAME	FORMULATION
primidone	MYSOLINE	250mg, 250mg/5ml

Maximum of 1.5G daily.
Children: maintenance — up to 2 years 250–500mg, 2–5 years 500–750mg, 6–9 years 750mg–1G, 9–12 years 750mg–1.5G. All daily.

CARBOXYLIC ACID DERIVATIVE

Category III drug.
Used in petit mal epilepsy particularly but may also be given in others.
Contraindications:
Active liver disease.

Effects:
General: drowsiness, lethargy, malaise.
Central nervous system: slurred speech, stammering, ataxia, tremor, coma, involuntary movements, twitching of face and limbs, increase in frequency of convulsions.
Psychological: confusion even progressing to stuporose states, hallucinations, increase in alertness, aggression, hyperactivity, behavioural deterioration, bad dreams.
Gastrointestinal: stomatitis, increase in appetite with consequent increase in weight, minor gastric irritation, nausea.
Liver dysfunction including hepatic failure (including deaths). Those most at risk are children under the age of 3, those with organic brain disease or severe convulsions associated with mental retardation.
In patients with a prior history of liver disease there should be liver investigations performed before starting treatment and during the first six months. These patients should have close clinical supervision.
Liver function tests may become abnormal anyway during treatment with this drug and such patients should be reassessed regularly with routine tests until they return to normal. Up to 50% of patients have some evidence of change in liver function.
Pancreatitis may develop and if abdominal pain occurs this diagnosis should be checked.
Endocrine: amenorrhoea.Skin: transient hair loss, change in hair colour or texture, rashes.
Blood disorders: thrombocytopenia, leucopenia.

CHEM NAME	TRADE NAME	FORMULATION
sodium valproate	EPILIM	100mg, 200mg, 500mg, 200/5ml

Usual maintenance 1–2G daily. Maximum 2.5G daily.
Children: under 20Kg, 20mg/Kg body-weight daily, over 20Kg initially 400mg daily. Maximum 40mg/Kg daily.

GABA ANALOGUE

Category III drug.
This is a very new drug and used for epilepsy not controlled satisfactorily by other anticonvulsants.

Precautions:
The elderly and those with renal impairment.
Effects:
General: drowsiness, fatigue.
Central nervous system: dizziness. Certain types of epilepsy (myoclonic) is exacerbated.
Psychological: nervousness, irritability, memory disturbances, excitation and agitation in children.
Special senses: visual disturbances.

CHEM NAME	TRADE NAME	FORMULATION
vigabatrin	SABRIL	500mg

4 daily increasing as needed. Maximum 8 daily.
Children: under 3 years not recommended, 3–9 years 2 initially, over 9 years as adult.

COMMENTS

Epilepsy is a difficult condition to treat because patients invariably take medication and society is very hostile to altered states of consciousness in general and epileptiform attacks specifically.

However, it is possible to help if care is taken and in selected cases. All the drugs have similar effects in suppressing the symptoms of change in consciousness, loss of consciousness and involuntary movements of the 'fit' and in this sense are depressant or sedating in nature.

The pathology is shifted through into the mental and/or emotional sphere with effects of sedation, drowsiness, confusion, irritability or paradoxical hyperactivity and deterioration of behaviour.

The danger with drug reduction is the risk of return of the fits. However in patients who have been fit-free for 2 years on medication drug withdrawal leads to reappearance of attacks in about 30%.[12] Clearly the exciting factor has now ended and the drugs are no longer necessary. Unfortunately you won't know which 30% until after reduction.

Many epileptics take a 'cocktail' of several drugs — especially in the more severe cases. In certain doses, combinations and situations they can also produce 'fits'. It is important to be aware of this particularly with multiple prescriptions.

Drugs which are stimulant in nature such as antidepressants and sympathomimetics may lead to worsening of epilepsy and so larger doses of anticonvulsants.

When dealing with an individual case do not be too overawed by the actual label of epilepsy. It merely describes a certain group of symptoms associated with EEG (electroencephalogram) changes. As such there are many different manifestations and severities. EEG changes are not particularly relevant to the alternative practitioner as they are probably very common — even in the 'normal' population. Concentrate on the clinical picture.

Once treatment is instituted and improvement begins drug reduction may begin (markers of improvement will have to be symptoms other than 'fits' in those whose attacks are controlled by drugs).

To minimise the risk of an epileptic attack reduction should be very slow, account should be taken of the patient's occupation and activities — particularly if involving driving, operating machinery and so on — and general stress levels.

It is important to involve the family so that they are supportive in this process.

Clearly, as drug withdrawal is underway the clinical situation will be less stable and so the patient should endeavour to relax, not pursue activities which are strenuous or stressful and generally lead a lifestyle which is not stimulating. In this way the risk of a 'fit' occurring is minimised. If a 'fit' does take place then the patient should take action at the first sign of this by lying down, keeping away from possible sources of injury, removing glasses and sharp objects.

How far it is possible to reduce dosage is dependent on each case and it is difficult to generalise. Certainly in cases where this is possible there is improved health, less side-effects and the possibility of a drug-free life.

11   ARTHRITIS

Non-Steroidal Anti-Inflammatory Agents (NSAID's)

These are commonly used in the treatment of all types of arthritis whether inflammatory in origin or not. Some varieties e.g. PONSTAN may be given for the pain of dysmenorrhoea.

People with acute strains of muscles or the back may also receive them although they are of dubious effectiveness even conventionally for this.

As a group they are similar in action to aspirin. They are used as first-line treatment in many types of arthritis, both inflammatory and degenerative, musculoskeletal pain of any cause, injury, backache and so on.

They are acidic in origin, have similar effects on the gastrointestinal tract, are in common use and lead to analgesic nephropathy.

The incidence of gastric lesions vary with the different formulations. The general incidence is 30% although indomethacin is at that level with the others ranging between 20–25%. Aspirin may produce erosions in up to 50% of patients.

They are closely related to each other and to aspirin and so there is often cross-sensitivity.

Aspirin is listed on page 210 (see analgesics) and is commonly used in many forms of arthritis.

The NSAID's as a group are commonly used in the treatment of arthritis of all types. They have similar actions and effects and I have summarised them together as much as possible. Any departures from this or additions are listed under the individual entry.

Contraindications:

History or evidence of peptic ulceration, ulcerative colitis, blood disorders, liver or kidney impairment.

Patients on long term treatment should be regularly reviewed.

Suppositories should not be used in those with inflammatory conditions of the anus, rectum and sigmoid colon.

Precautions:

NSAID's can precipitate bronchospasm in patients with asthma or allergic disease.

Patients with impaired hearing should have regular tests of hearing function.

Eye examinations should be performed if visual disturbances occur.

All patients receiving long-term treatment with NSAID's should be monitored by means of renal, hepatic function and blood counts. Some patients may develop gross evidence of renal impairment. These include the elderly, those taking diuretics and those with impaired renal function, heart failure and liver dysfunction.

Genitourinary tract symptoms of dysuria, cystitis, haematuria, nephritis and the nephrotic syndrome may occur. Some patients have required dialysis and corticosteroid treatment.

Liver function tests become abnormal in 15% of patients. If these tests show a worsening of the results then the drug should be stopped since severe hepatic reactions including jaundice and fatal hepatitis have occurred.

Caution in patients with hypertension and impaired cardiac function because some develop oedema an effect.

Effects:

General: drowsiness, fatigue, lymphadenopathy, fever.

Allergic reactions: these take two forms. Firstly there may be the development of wheezing (asthma) with rhinitis and nasal polyps and secondly there may be urticaria with oedema.

Cardiovascular: palpitations, rapid heart rate, pulmonary oedema, peripheral oedema, high blood pressure, low blood pressure, congestive cardiac failure, chest pain.

Respiratory: breathlessness, cough, wheezing (due to development of fibrosing alveolitis).

Central nervous system: headache, dizziness, tinnitus, deafness, vertigo, tremor, convulsions, trigeminal neuralgia.

Psychological: confusion, insomnia, depression, nervousness, personality change, hallucinations, mood alterations, dream abnormalities.

Gastrointestinal: nausea, vomiting, anorexia, metallic taste in mouth, burning tongue, constipation or diarrhoea, flatulence, indigestion or heartburn, development of oesophageal stricture, bleeding and peptic ulceration, development or worsening of inflammatory bowel disease (Crohn's disease and ulcerative colitis), blood in the stool on laboratory testing. Pancreatitis. Hepatitis with or without jaundice or other abnormalities of liver function. Bleeding may be precipitated in diverticular disease.

There is known way to prevent or reduce the occurrence of gastrointestinal problems although some formulations just released also contain anti-ulcer agents. This seems to be unable to prevent such problems.

Suppositories may lead to the development of rectal inflammation, swelling, pain and bleeding.

Urogenital: renal insufficiency, haematuria, nephrotic syndrome, dysuria, cystitis, haematuria.

Endocrine: gynaecomastia, breast enlargement and tenderness, vaginal bleeding, hyperglycaemia, glycosuria.

Blood disorders: anaemia, haemolytic anaemia, leucopenia, thrombocytopenia, aplastic anaemia.

Skin: rashes such as nettle rash, eczema, photosensitivity. Alopecia, increased sweating, pruritus.

Special senses: impaired hearing, blurred vision, double vision, epistaxis, retinal changes, corneal opacities.

BENZOTRIAZINE

CHEM NAME	TRADE NAME	FORMULATION
azapropazone	RHEUMOX	300mg, 600mg

Adults: 1.2G daily.
Elderly: 600mg daily, increasing up to maximum of 900mg daily if renal function is normal.
Not for children.
This drug is related to phenylbutazone and has very similar effects although does not seem to affect the blood.

SALICYLATE-PARACETAMOL
Contraindications:
It should not be given to children under the age of 12 because of the link between aspirin and Reye's syndrome.
Precautions:
Patients should be warned not to also take aspirin or paracetamol.

CHEM NAME	TRADE NAME	FORMULATION
benorylate	BENORAL	750mg, 4G/10ml, 2G sachets.

Tablets 2 three times daily or 5–10ml twice daily or 1–2 sachets twice daily.
Not for children.

PHENYLACETIC ACID

CHEM NAME	TRADE NAME	FORMULATION
diclofenac	RHUMALGAN	25mg, 50mg
	VALENAC	25mg, 50mg
	VOLRAMAN	25mg, 50mg
	VOLTAROL	25mg, 50mg

75–150mg daily.
Children: over 1 year 1–3mg/Kg daily.

	TRADE NAME	FORMULATION
	VOLTAROL RETARD	100mg sustained-release

1 once daily.
Not for children.

	TRADE NAME	FORMULATION
	VOLTAROL SUPPOSITORIES	100mg

1 at night.

	TRADE NAME	FORMULATION
	VOLTAROL PAED. SUPPOSITORIES	12.5mg

Children: 1–3mg/Kg daily.
In addition to the above, this drug may cause agranulocytosis and granulocytopenia.

PYRANOCARBOXYLATE

CHEM NAME	TRADE NAME	FORMULATION
etodolac	LODINE	200mg, 300mg

200mg twice daily. Maximum 600mg daily.
Not for children.

PROPIONIC ACID

CHEM NAME	TRADE NAME	FORMULATION
fenbufen	LEDERFEN	300mg, 450mg
	LEDERFEN F	450mg

900mg daily.
Not for children.

CHEM NAME	TRADE NAME	FORMULATION
fenoprofen	FENOPRON	300mg, 600mg
	PROGESIC	200mg

300–600mg three or four times daily. Maximum 3G daily.

Not for children.
In addition to the above, this drug may cause pancytopenia,
granulocytopenia, agranulocytosis, renal failure.

flurbiprofen	FROBEN	50mg, 100mg, 100mg suppository

150–200mg daily. Maximum 300mg daily.
Not for children.

	FROBEN SR	200mg sustained-release

1 daily.
Not for children.
This is the most toxic of this group with the elderly experiencing
adverse effects in 80% of cases.

ibuprofen	APSIFEN	200mg, 400mg
	APSIFEN F	600mg
	ARTHROFEN	
	BRUFEN	200mg, 400mg, 600mg, 100mg/5ml
	EBUFAC	400mg
	JUNIFEN	100mg/5ml
	LIDIFEN	200mg, 400mg
	MOTRIN	200mg, 400mg, 600mg, 800mg
	PAXOFEN	200mg, 400mg, 600mg

1200–1800mg daily. Maximum 2400mg daily.
Children: usually 20mg/Kg daily. Dose should not exceed 500mg daily
for those less than 30Kg.

	FENBID SPANSULE	300mg sustained-release

Maintenance 1–2 twice daily.
Not for children.
This drug may cause, in addition to the above, agranulocytosis and
pancytopenia (may be fatal).

ketoprofen	ALRHEUMAT	50mg
	ORUDIS	50mg, 100mg (suppositories)
	ORUVAIL	100mg, 200mg

100–200mg daily.
Suppositories 1 at night supplemented during the day with capsules
if necessary.
Not for children.
This drug is very similar in its actions to ibuprofen.

naproxen	ARTHROSIN	
	LARAFLEX	250mg, 500mg
	NAPROSYN	250mg, 500mg, 250mg/10ml, 500mg sachet, 500mg suppository.

VALROX

500mg–1G daily.
Children: under 5 years not recommended, 5–12 years 10mg/Kg daily.
Suppository, 1 at night. If necessary another suppository or 500mg
orally in the morning. Not for children.

SYNFLEX   275mg

Acute sprain/strain: Over 16 years 2 twice daily.
Not for children.
In addition to the above this drug may cause impotence, failure of
ejaculation, tinnitus and acne (in women who take it for
dysmenorrhoea).

tiaprofenic acid	SURGAM	200mg, 300mg
	SURGAM SA	300mg sustained-release

600mg daily.
Not for children.

INDOLE
Contraindications:
Nasal polyps associated with attacks of allergic oedema.
Precautions:
Psychiatric disorder, epilepsy, Parkinson's disease (they may all
be exacerbated).
The drug may mask the signs and symptoms of infection.

CHEM NAME	TRADE NAME	FORMULATION
indomethacin	ARTRACIN	25mg, 50mg
	FLEXIN CONTINUS	75mg controlled-release
	IMBRILON	25mg, 50mg, 100mg (suppositories)
	INDOCID	25mg, 50mg, 25mg/5ml, 100mg (suppositories)
	INDOCID R	75mg sustained-release
	INDOLAR SR	75mg sustained-release
	INDOMOD	25mg, 75mg controlled-release

50–75mg daily increasing as necessary. Maximum 200mg daily.
Suppositories — 1 at night plus one morning if necessary.
Not for children.
This drug , in addition to the above, causes headache in up to 60% of
patients which is usually migrainous in nature. It may also lead
togranulocytopenia and agranulocytosis.

sulindac   CLINORIL   100mg, 200mg
200mg twice daily.
Not for children.
In addition to the above, this drug may cause bizarre behaviour and
paranoia, agranulocytosis, bone marrow aplasia, congestive heart
failure and palpitations.

FENAMATE

CHEM NAME	TRADE NAME	FORMULATION
mefenamic acid	DYSMAN	250mg
	PONSTAN	250mg, 50mg/5ml
	PONSTAN FORTE	500mg

500mg three times daily.
Children: under 6 months not recommended, 6 months–1 year 5ml, 2–4
years 10ml, 5–8 years 15ml, 9–12 years 20ml. All three times daily for
not more than 7 days.
Also used in dysmenorrhoea.
This drug may cause, in addition to the above, agranulocytosis,
neutropenia, steatorrhoea and abdominal distension.

ALKANONE

CHEM NAME	TRADE NAME	FORMULATION
nabumetone	RELIFLEX	500mg

2 daily at night. In more severe cases an additional 1–2 tablets in the
morning.
Elderly: 1–2 daily.
Not for children.

PYRAZONE

This is only used for ankylosing spondylitis where other
treatments have not been effective.
Contraindications:
History of peptic ulcer, gastrointestinal haemorrhage or blood
disease, if there is severe cardiac, hepatic or renal insufficiency,
oedema, hypertension or thyroid disease.

Precautions:
Now only available to hospital prescribers because of the danger of aplastic anaemia. This leads to death in 50% of those affected and has caused over 1100 deaths to date.

The elderly are particularly prone to side-effects.

Care with a history of dyspepsia.

All patients should have regular blood counts and the drug stopped if there is any decrease in platelet, white or red blood cell counts.

Treatment should also be stopped if symptoms suggestive of these appear such as bruising, fever, sore throat, rash, mouth ulceration and so on. Patients should be specifically told to report such symptoms.

Oedema may occur and this should be taken into account in patients with hypertension or cardiovascular disease.

Systemic lupus erythematosus may be aggravated.

It may also lead to parotitis, corneal damage, retinal haemorrhage, blindness.

CHEM NAME	TRADE NAME	FORMULATION
phenylbutazone	BUTACOTE	100mg, 200mg

Hospital use only.
Usually 200–300mg daily.
Elderly: always use the minimum effective dose.

OXICAM

CHEM NAME	TRADE NAME	FORMULATION
piroxicam	FELDENE	10mg, 20mg, 20mg suppository

20mg daily.
Musculo-skeletal disorders, 20mg daily for 7–14 days.
Not for children.

tenoxicam	MOBIFLEX	20mg

1 daily.
Not for children.

ACETIC ACID DERIVATIVE

CHEM NAME	TRADE NAME	FORMULATION
tolmetin	TOLECTIN	200mg, 400mg

Maintenance 600–1800mg daily.
Children: 20–25mg/Kg daily.
10% of patients who take this drug have to stop it because of its effects. In addition to the above, this drug may cause hearing loss and renal failure.

Second Line Drugs

The following are used as second-line in inflammatory arthritides such as rheumatoid arthritis.

These are much more powerful with more severe side-effects.

GOLD SALT

These are used in the treatment of rheumatoid arthritis where NSAID's have been found to be ineffective or of limited use. They may need to be taken for 3–6 months of treatment before a response and can only relieve the inflammatory symptoms, they cannot reverse joint destruction.

Contraindications:

Pulmonary fibrosis, necrotizing enterocolitis, exfoliative dermatitis or severe blood diseases, progressive renal disease, severe active hepatic disease and in systemic lupus erythematosus.

Precautions:

Renal or hepatic impairment, inflammatory bowel disease, rash or if there is a history of bone marrow depression.

Full blood count and tests for urinary protein should be performed before therapy starts and at least monthly thereafter. Patients who have gastrointestinal symptoms, rash, pruritus, stomatitis or metallic taste in the mouth should also be closely monitored as the drug may have to be reduced in dosage or withdrawn.

Before treatment begins patients should be informed of the effects. They should be specifically told to report itching, rash, metallic taste, sore throat or tongue, mouth ulceration, easy bruising, purpura, epistaxis, bleeding gums, menorrhagia or diarrhoea.

Women of child-bearing age should practice effective contraception during treatment and for at least 6 months after since this drug can cause foetal abnormalities. Patients should be warned of this.

Effects:

The injected form may lead within a few minutes to the development of weakness, fainting, hypotension, rapid heart rate, palpitations, sweating. This may be followed by a heart attack or stroke.

Respiratory: pulmonary fibrosis leading to breathlessness , dry cough, weakness and malaise.. Chest X Ray should be performed at least annually. This syndrome develops after a few weeks or months of treatment usually.

General: increased incidence of herpes zoster. Systemic lupus erythematosus. Fever.

Gastrointestinal: nausea, diarrhoea, loose stools, stomatitis, oral mucous membrane reactions, taste disturbances including a metallic taste. Changes in liver function, jaundice.

One patient in twenty cannot tolerate RIDAURA because of diarrhoea.

Ulcerative enterocolitis can occur (life-threatening). Mmetallic taste can occur.

Central nervous system: peripheral neuropathy.

Psychological: insomnia.

Skin (effects seen in 25%): rashes, itching, alopecia, eczema, urticaria, photosensitivity. The drug is stopped if these become severe and in some recovery does not occur.

Urogenital: proteinuria, nephrotic syndrome, haematuria.

Blood: agranulocytosis, thrombocytopenia (causing bleeding), granulocytopenia, pancytopenia, eosinophilia, leucopenia. Regular blood checks should be made.

CHEM NAME	TRADE NAME	FORMULATION
auranofin	RIDAURA	3mg

6mg daily continued for a minimum of 3–6 months. If response is inadequate increase to maximum of 9mg daily. Discontinue after a further 3 months if response remains inadequate.
Not for children.

sodium aurothiomalate	MYOCRISIN	injection

Given by injection at weekly intervals.

AMINOQUINOLINE

This is a quinine derivative used as a second-line in the treatment of rheumatoid arthritis.

Contraindications:

Certain pre-existing eye conditions (disease of the macular).

Precautions:

All patients should have an opthalmological examination before starting treatment. They should be repeated every 6 months. The drug must be stopped immediately if any defect develops.

Some blurring of vision is common at the start of treatment due to changes in focussing and patients should be specifically warned of this especially in relation to driving and operating machinery.

Caution in cases of allergic or eye reactions to other drugs, renal or hepatic disease, those who take drugs known to affect the liver or kidney, those with severe gastrointestinal, neurological or blood disorders.

Regular blood counts should be taken.

Effects:

Central nervous system: muscle weakness, vertigo, tinnitus, nerve deafness, headache, peripheral neuritis.

Psychological: nervousness, emotional upsets, psychosis, depression, agitation, aggressiveness, confusion, personality changes.

Gastrointestinal: nausea, diarrhoea, anorexia, abdominal cramps, vomiting.

Blood: bone marrow depression, leucopenia, agranulocytosis.

Skin: rashes, depigmentation of skin or hair, hair loss.

Special senses: eye problems are the most important including retinal changes and corneal opacities (these may be experienced as haloes, blurring of vision or photophobia).

CHEM NAME	TRADE NAME	FORMULATION
hydroxy-chloroquine	PLAQUENIL	200mg

Maintenance 1–2 daily. Maximum 6.5mg/Kg body-weight daily. Discontinue treatment after 6 months if no improvement.

PENICILLIN DERIVATIVE

This a second-line agent used in the treatment of rheumatoid arthritis.

Contraindications:
Penicillin allergy, lupus erythematosus, thrombocytopenia, agranulocytosis.

Precautions:
Blood counts should be performed and renal function assessed before treatment begins. Blood counts should be monitored regularly (monthly) along with urinalysis for detection of blood and protein.

Care should be exercised in those with renal insufficiency or in patients who also take drugs which may damage the bone marrow.

Because of the occurrence of polyneuropathy it is wise for the patient to also take Vitamin B6 at the same time to prevent its development.

Effects:
General: fever.

Allergic reactions: a syndrome may appear of haemturia, urticaria, itching, oedema, lymphadenopathy, joint pain, fever and eosinophilia.

Respiratory: recurrent respiratory tract infections.

Central nervous system: polyneuropathy.

Gastrointestinal: nausea, vomiting, anorexia, loss of taste, stomatitis, hepatitis, pancreatitis.

Urogenital: proteinuria in 30% (urine should be checked weekly at first and after each increase in dosage, thereafter monthly), haematuria, nephrotic syndrome.

Skin: rash.

Blood: thrombocytopenia (10% — with some fall in platelet seen in 75%), leucopenia, agranulocytosis, aplastic anaemia, anaemia, haemolytic anaemia.

There is a suggestion in some sources that this drug may be implicated in the development of leukaemia.

Drug induced systemic lupus erythematosus, conditions resembling myasthenia gravis and rheumatoid arthritis.

CHEM NAME	TRADE NAME	FORMULATION
penicillamine	DISTAMINE	25mg, 125mg, 250mg
	PENDRAMINE	125mg, 250mg

Maintenance 500–750mg. Maximum 1.5G daily.
Elderly: 50–125mg daily increasing to maintenance. Maximum 1G daily.

SALICYLATE-SULPHONAMIDE

This a second-line drug for the treatment of rheumatoid arthritis. It is also used in ulcerative colitis (see page 254 for details).

CHEM NAME	TRADE NAME	FORMULATION
sulphasalazine	SALAZOPYRIN EN	500mg
Maximum of 6 daily.		
Not for children.		

COMMENTS

A further category used as the third-line in inflammatory arthritides are the corticosteroids (see page 258). These drugs may be used for osteoarthritis, tennis elbow, tendon problems and the like in injectable form. Patients may have a joint injected several times with such a drug.

Fourth-line drugs are the immunosuppressants. They are not commonly seen and only used in extremely severe forms of the disease. Conventional medical advice is needed when these drugs are taken.

Table of drugs used in order of increasing severity:

> CATEGORY I
> - analgesic — symptomatic
> - non-steroidal anti-inflammatory agent — symptomatic
>
> CATEGORY II
> - analgesic — prophylactic
> - non-steroidal anti-inflammatory agent — prophylactic
> - second-line drug — gold, penicillamine or quinine
>
> CATEGORY III
> - corticosteroids — injected locally
> - corticosteroids — oral
>
> CATEGORY V
> - immunosuppressant (not included in this book).

Complete one drug at a time in sequence. Withdrawal symptoms mainly centre around the joints with a flareup of swelling, pain and stiffness.

However, when second-line agents or stronger are used in cases of rheumatoid arthritis, for example, withdrawal may lead to constitutional symptoms in keeping with that disease such as fever, anorexia, tiredness and so on.

In rheumatoid arthritis which is an example of a deep, degenerative disease of the immune system, treatment will necessarily be prolonged and so there is plenty of time to reduce dosages.

Gout

In orthodox medicine this condition is considered due to a raised level of uric acid in the blood which is then deposited in the joints. The result is an extremely painful inflammatory arthritis. This mainly involves the first metatarsophalangeal joint although others may be affected in time.

The treatment is usually with a combination of drugs — non-steroidal inflammatory agents as used in other types of arthritis and drugs which lower uric acid levels.

When faced with this disease treat as any other arthritis but bear in mind that the group of xanthine oxidase inhibitors and uricosurics are given prophylactically. Therefore reduce these first and do so slowly when appropriate since with rising uric acid levelsthere may be brief flare-ups of gout. With effective treatment these will be temporary as patients improve.

XANTHINE OXIDASE INHIBITOR

Category II drug.

This drug is effective because it interferes with the production of uric acid.

Contraindications:

If treatment is begun during an attack of gout it can be worsened.

Precautions:

Reduced dosage is given in severe renal or hepatic disease.

Effects:

General: acute attack of gout. (NSAID should be given at the same time for the first month).

Gastrointestinal: nausea, vomiting, recurrent haematemesis, hepatitis.

Blood: reduced numbers of blood cells (usually transient).

Skin: pruritus, rashes (these reactions necessitate the immediate cessation of treatment).

Skin reactions with fever, enlargement of lymph glands, joint pains and eosinophilia. These symptoms are suggestive of a severe allergic reaction. Allopurinol must be stopped suddenly if this occurs and corticosteroids are usually given.

Other reactions which have occurred during treatment but are not known to be definitely related to the drug include:

General: fever, malaise, tiredness.

Cardiovascular: angina, hypertension, slow heart rate, oedema, raised blood lipid levels.

Gastrointestinal: taste in mouth, stomatitis, change in bowel habit, hepatitis, changes in liver function.

Psychological: sleepiness, depression.

Central nervous system: headache, vertigo, ataxia, paralysis, parasthesiae, neuropathy.

Endocrine: diabetes mellitus.

Urogenital: uraemia, haematuria, impotence, nocturnal emission, infertility.

Special senses: visual disturbances, cataract.

Skin: alopecia, discoloured hair, boils.

CHEM NAME	TRADE NAME	FORMULATION
allopurinol	ALULINE	100mg, 300mg
	CAPLENAL	100mg, 300mg
	COSURIC	100, 300mg
	HAMARIN	100mg, 300mg
	XANTHOMAX	100mg, 300mg
	ZYLORIC	100mg, 300mg

Maintenance of 200–600mg daily.

URICOSURIC

This group of drugs increases urinary excretion of uric acid. Therefore there is a risk of development of urate renal stones. Patients must be told to avoid dehydration and to maintain fluid intake.

SULPHINPYRAZONE

Category II drug.

Contraindications:

Active peptic ulcer, severe hepatic disease. Do not use aspirin if taking long term.

Precautions:
Care must be taken in those with impaired renal function, history of peptic ulcer, asthma preciptitated by aspirin.
Renal function must be checked regularly as well as blood counts to monitor blood cell levels..
Effects:
General: acute attack of gout.
Gastrointestinal: mild disturbances, bleeding.
Urogenital: impaired renal function.
Blood: disturbances in blood cell production.
Skin: rash.

CHEM NAME	TRADE NAME	FORMULATION
sulphinpyrazone	ANTURAN	100mg, 200mg

Maintenance is with the lowest dose effective. 600mg given in the first few weeks is reduced as much as possible.

PROBENECID

Category II drug.
Contraindications:
Acute attack of gout, history of blood diseases. Aspirin must not be given at the same time.
Precautions:
Care must be taken in those with a history of peptic ulcer.
Effects:
General: fever, anaphylaxis.
Gastrointestinal: nausea, vomiting, anorexia, sore gums, hepatic necrosis.
Central nervous system: headache, dizziness.
Blood: anaemia, haemolytic anaemia, aplastic anaemia.
Urogenital: frequent urination, nephrotic syndrome, urate stones, renal colic.
Skin: dermatitis, pruritus, flushing.

CHEM NAME	TRADE NAME	FORMULATION
probenecid	BENEMID	500mg

2 daily.

12 ENDOCRINE SYSTEM

CORTICOSTEROIDS

These are normal substances in the body produced by the adrenal glands. They have many functions concerned with responses to shock, infection and stressful situations as well as having a role in carbohydrate metabolism.

Clinically they are used primarily for their anti-inflammatory actions. We see their use in conditions featuring inflammation (not infection) particularly in those diseases with no known cause or due to autoimmune factors. Examples of these are rheumatoid arthritis, ulcerative colitis, eczema, asthma, collagen disorders such as systemic lupus erythematosus.

The following refers to corticosteroids as a group. Many dangers of these drugs are due to their ability to mask inflammatory processes. Therefore infections worsen dramatically and problems such as peptic ulcer may exist with few or no symptoms.

Contraindications:
Herpes simplex and TB.

Precautions:
Caution with active peptic ulcer, acute glomerulonephritis, myasthenia gravis, osteoporosis, fresh intestinal anastomoses, diverticulitis, thrombophlebitis, psychological disturbances, pregnancy, local or systemic infections.

With chronic use it is advisable to perform faecal occult blood tests and barium meal or gastroscopy because of the danger of upper gastrointestinal lesions.

Effects:
The severity and number of effects seen will depend upon the dosage used and the duration of treatment. If corticosteroids are used for replacement in Addison's disease then adverse effects are unusual.

General: fatigue, moon face, buffalo hump, osteoporosis, spontaneous fractures, diminished immune response, aggravation of infection,

Cardiovascular: thrombo-embolism, high blood pressure, oedema. Central nervous system: raised intracranial pressure, headache, vertigo, convulsions.

Psychological: psychological disturbances, insomnia, behavioural and personality changes, nervousness, insomnia, euphoria, mood swings, manic states, depression, paranoia, psychotic episodes.

Syndromes of confusion, disorientation, apathy and memory loss are seen.

Gastrointestinal: nausea, anorexia, indigestion, gastrointestinal haemorrhage, peptic ulcer, pancreatitis. Crohn's disease and ulcerative colitis may worsen.

Endocrine: high blood sugar,

Urogenital: renal stones. Menstrual disorders are common, amenorrhoea.

Inhibition of ovulation occurs at high dosage. Reduced sperm count and motility.

Skin: facial flushing, striae, acne, purpura, hirsutism, atrophic changes, bruising.

Blood disorders: leucocytosis with fall in eosinophils and lymphocytes.

CHEM NAME	TRADE NAME	FORMULATION
betamethasone	BETNELAN	0.5mg
	BETNESOL	0.5mg

0.5–5mg daily Reduce for maintenance to minimum effective dose. Children: under 1 year not recommended. 1–7 years quarter to half of adult dose, 7–12 years half to three quarters of adult dose.

cortisone	CORTELAN	25mg
	CORTISTAB	5mg, 25mg
	CORTISYL	25mg

12.5–300mg daily.
This drug is used for inflammatory disorders as well as for hormone replacement in cases of Addison's disease.

dexamethasone	DECADRON	0.5mg

Maintenance 0.5–1.5mg daily.

hydrocortisone	CORLAN	2.5mg pellet

Chewed or sucked in cases of apthous ulceration.

	HYDROCORTISTAB	20mg
	HYDROCORTONE	10mg, 20mg

10–30mg daily.
This drug is used for inflammatory disorders as well as for hormone replacement in cases of Addison's disease.

methyl- prednisolone	MEDRONE	2mg, 4mg, 16mg

Varying doses are given according to the condition.

- ulcerative colitis — 16–60mg
- rheumatoid arthritis
  severe — 12–16mg
  moderately severe — 8–12mg
  moderate — 4–8mg

- SLE — 20–96mg
- allergic disease, asthma, rhinitis and dermatitis up to 40mg.

All daily doses.

These can only be a guide because in some severe cases you will see these doses exceeded.

prednisolone	DELTACORTRIL	2.5mg, 5mg
	DELTASTAB	1mg, 5mg
	PRECORTISYL	1mg, 5mg
	PRECORTISYL FORTE	25mg
	PREDNESOL	5mg
	SINTISONE	5mg

Dose varies according to the condition. In general a fairly high dose is initially given then reduced to the lowest maintenance possible. The final dose will depend upon the severity of the condition.
The following can only be a guide:

- allergic and skin disease — 5–15mg daily.
- collagen disorders — 20–30mg daily.
- rheumatoid arthritis — 10–15mg daily initially.
- blood disorders and lymphoma — 60mg daily.

For example, 7mg a day long-term in an asthmatic would be a fairly high dose.

Children: under 1 year not recommended, 1–7 years quarter to half of adult dose, 7–12 years half to three quarters of adult dose.

| prednisone | DECORTISYL | 5mg |

Maintenance of 5–20mg daily depending on the condition.
Children: under 1 year not recommended, 1–7 years quarter to half of adult dose, 7–12 years half to three quarters of adult dose.

| triamcinolone | LEDERCORT | 2mg, 4mg |

Varying doses are given according to the condition.

- rheumatoid arthritis — maintenance of 2–16mg daily.
- systemic lupus erythematosus — maintenance of 3–30mg daily.
- skin conditions — maintenance of 1–2mg daily.

These can only be a guide because in severe cases you will see these doses exceeded.

COMMENTS

These drugs are extremely powerful as evidenced by the list of effects. They will produce a situation similar to Cushing's syndrome. They are very powerful suppressants and often rapidly antidote treatment with alternative medicine. They are to be considered in Category III as detailed on page 18.

When dealing with these agents it is important to consider:

- dose
- duration of the medication
- condition for which given
- other treatment
- patient's energetic state

Corticosteroids are very depleting and some people who take them for a long time are in such a state when they present for treatment that little can be done.

If the use of corticosteroids has been long term, the patient's energy weak and the clinical picture unclear then it may be better not to take the case.

If the use of corticosteroids has been long term but the patient's energy is stronger and the clinical picture is clear then diagnosis and treatment can be initiated. You may have to treat more often. Some homoeopaths use more frequent administration of low potency remedies. However alternative treatment can still be effective even 'through' the drug.

If the use of corticosteroids is not current then the case can be taken as usual and treatment begun. It is common experience that patients who have received these drugs in the past — whether for rheumatoid arthritis, injections for tennis elbow, creams for eczema and so on — are more difficult to treat. Treatment is longer and aggravations are more severe. However, such patients can be usually be treated quite successfully.

What to do with a case where corticosteroids are currently being taken? The problem lies in the fact that their action is severely suppressive and so reduction in dosage often leads to a flareup in the symptoms. It is difficult to 'see' the true clinical picture. You may have to treat more often, homoeopaths may have to use low potency remedies but treatment can still be effective even 'through' the drug.

The same rules apply whether the drug is administered orally, inhaled, applied to the skin, used as an enema and so on. Treat the patient until an improvement occurs. Bear in mind the original diagnosis since exacerbations may be potentially serious.

Reduce the dose slowly e.g. if prednisolone 6mg daily is being taken in a case of asthma the reduction would be around 1mg every three to four weeks. It should certainly be no quicker than this.

The corticosteroids listed above are of differing strengths. The equivalents to 1mg of prednisolone are:

- 0.12mg betamethasone
- 5mg cortisone
- 0.15mg dexamethasone
- 4mg hydrocortisone
- 0.8mg methylprednisolone
- 0.8mg triamcinolone

In terms of prednisolone:

1mg daily is a low dose
5mg daily is a moderate dose
10mg or more daily is a high dose

Allow patients to use the other drugs they may be taking such as bronchodilators in asthma, non-steroidal anti-inflammatory drugs in rheumatoid arthritis and so on. These will support the patient whilst the powerful corticosteroids are reduced.

When the corticosteroids are eventually stopped then it is possible to start on the less powerful drugs.

Sex Hormones

These are the hormones normally secreted by the sex organs — testis and ovary. There are small amounts of androgens and oestrogens also produced by the adrenal glands.

They are responsible for the development of the secondary sex characteristics. In women their cyclical release governs the menstrual cycle.

Clinically female hormones are used for contraception, replacement therapy after the menopause, acne in young females, hormone-sensitive tumours, premenstrual syndrome, infertility, habitual abortion (miscarriage), menstrual disorders, endometriosis.

Male hormones are used for underactivity of testicular function. Of course the anabolic steroids are used by some athletes to build muscle bulk and may sometimes be given to men for underweight.

CHEM NAME	TRADE NAME	FORMULATION

GONADOTROPHIN RELEASE INHIBITOR

Indications:
This drug is used in the treatment of endometriosis, benign breast disease, menorrhagia and premenstrual syndrome by suppressing pituitary function.

Contraindications:
Pregnant women. Lactation.

Precautions:
This drug should not be relied upon for contraception. Patients should use a non-hormonal method of contraception.
Caution with cardiac or renal impairment and migraine because fluid retention may occur.
Caution also in liver impairment.
This drug may exacerbate diabetes mellitus.

Effects:
General: fluid retention, backache, muscle cramps, tiredness.
Cardiovascular: hypertension.
Central nervous system: headache, vertigo, dizziness.
Psychological: nervousness, emotional lability, depression, anxiety.
Gastrointestinal: nausea, weight gain.
Endocrine: voice changes (deepening), reduction in breast size, clitoral hypertrophy.
Skin: acne, oily skin, mild hirsutism, flushing, rashes, hair loss.

CHEM NAME	TRADE NAME	FORMULATION
danazol	DANOL	200mg
	DANOL–½	100mg

Usually 200–800mg daily.
Endometriosis: initially 400mg daily.
Benign breast disease: initially 300mg daily.
Menorrhagia/Premenstrual syndrome: 200mg daily.
Treatment continues without interruption.

OESTROGEN

A normal female sex hormone produced mainly by the ovary particularly in the first half of the menstrual cycle.

The actions of these can be generally summarised as given below.

Contraindications:

Pregnancy, acute or chronic liver disease, severe cardiac or renal disease, history of thrombosis, history of severe disturbances of liver function, jaundice or general itching during a previous pregnancy, in the presence of hormone-dependent disorders or tumours of the uterus or breast, undiagnosed abnormal genital bleeding, otosclerosis.

Warnings:

There is an increased risk of endometrial carcinoma with treatment for over 1 year when oestrogens are given alone.

There is an increase in gall bladder disease when this agent is taken.

Blood pressure should be monitored at regular intervals.

Diabetic patients should be carefully monitored.

Caution in cerebral vascular or coronary artery disease.

Precautions:

Epilepsy, migraine, asthma, renal and cardiac impairment may be affected by the side-effect of fluid retention.

Diseases such as multiple sclerosis, epilepsy, otosclerosis may deteriorate during treatment.

Medication should be stopped if jaundice or thrombosis develops at least until the cause is determined.

Contraception should be provided by non-hormonal methods.

Uterine fibroids may increase in size and the symptoms of endometriosis exacerbated.

Caution in hyperthyroidism.

Effects:

General: epistaxis.

Cardiovascular: thrombophlebitis, high blood pressure.

Central nervous system: headaches, dizziness, vertigo, chorea, migraine.

Psychological: depression, changes in libido.

Gastrointestinal: dyspepsia, flatulence, nausea, vomiting, abdominal pain and bloating, weight gain, jaundice.

Benign liver tumours.

Urogenital: breakthrough bleeding, spotting, change in menstrual flow, endometrial carcinoma, dysmenorrhoea, premenstrual-like syndrome, amenorrhoea during and after

treatment, increase in size of uterine fibroids, vaginal thrush, change in cervical erosion, change in degree of cervical secretion, cystitis-like syndrome.
Breasts: tenderness, enlargement, secretion.
Skin: urticaria and other rashes, general pruritus, loss of scalp hair, hirsutism. There have been suggestions that oestrogen may be linked to the formation of malignant melanomas.
Special senses: intolerance of contact lenses.

CHEM NAME	TRADE NAME	FORMULATION
dinoestrol	ORTHO-Dinoestrol	0.01% cream

Maintenance 1 applicator dose one to three times per week.
Used for atrophic conditions of the vagina after the menopause.

mestranol	MENOPHASE	

With the addition of a progestogen — norethisterone. There are varying doses in phases of 5, 8, 2, 3, 6 and 4 tablets to be taken over the 28 days.
One daily without a break.
This drug is used for HRT around the menopause.

oestradiol	ESTRADERM	25mcg, 50mcg, 100mcg skin patches (dose per 24 hours)

New patch every 3–4 days. Dose depends on response.

	PROGYNOVA	1mg, 2mg

Initially 1mg daily for 21 days then at least 7 tablet-free days.
Higher strength only used when necessary.

	OESTRADIOL IMPLANTS	25mg, 50mg 100mg

These are implanted surgically at intervals of 6 months or so for HRT around the menopause.

	ESTRAPAK	50mcg skin patch with 1mg norethisterone tabs.

A combination of oestrogen and a progestogen.
New patch every 3–4 days. One tablet daily day 5 to day 26 of each 28 day oestrogen replacement.

	CYCLO-PROGYNOVA	1mg, 2mg

A combination of oestrogen and a progesterone.
11 days of oestradiol followed by 10 day of oestradiol with levonorgestrel.
One daily of the oestradiol for eleven days then ten days of the combined tablets followed by seven tablet free days.
Start on day 5 of the menses (if present) with the 1mg pack. Increase to the 2mg pack if required.

TRISEQUENS
A combination of oestrogen and a progestogen.
A sequence of 28 days cycle of treatment with varying strengths of oestradiol, oestriol and norethisterone.
1 daily without a break starting day 5 of the menses or arbitrarily if no menses.

oestriol	ORTHO-GYNEST	0.5mg pessary, 0.01% cream

Maintenance 1 pessary or 1 applicatorful twice weekly.

	OVESTIN	0.25mg tabs., 0.1% cream

1–2 tablets daily.
Cream: maintenance 1 applicator dose twice a week. Assess every 2–3 months.

	HORMONIN	0.27mg with oestrone, oestradiol

½–2 daily.
A mixture of oestrogens.

oestrogens	PREMARIN	0.625mg, 1.25mg, 2.5mg (conjugated)

Menopause, usually 0.625mg daily for 21 days starting on day 5 of menses or arbitrarily if absent, then 7 tablet-free days.

	PREMARIN CREAM	cream

1–2G via applicator daily for 3 weeks then one weeks rest.

	PREMPAK-C	0.625mgx28 tabs., 1.25x28 tabs., norgestrel 0.15mgx12

A mixture of an oestrogen and a progesterone.
One 0.625mg or 1.25mg tablet daily. After 16 days also take norgestrel for 12 days. Start day 1 of menses or arbitrarily.

piperazine oestrone sulphate	HARMOGEN	1.5mg

1–3 daily for three to four weeks then five to seven tablet free days.

stilboestrol	TAMPOVAGAN	0.5mg with lactic acid as pessary

2 intravaginally at night.

PROGESTOGEN

A normal female sex hormone produced mainly by the ovary particularly during the second half of the menstrual cycle.
The actions of these can be generally summarised as below.

Contraindications:
Existing thrombophlebitis, thrombosis, cerebral vascular disease, myocardial infarction or a past history of these disorders. Also excluded are patients with impaired liver function, known or suspected carcinoma of the breast, hormone-dependent tumours, pregnancy and undiagnosed abnormal genital bleeding.

Precautions:
Examination of the pelvis (vaginal examination), breast and blood pressure should be performed before this drug is prescribed and they should be repeated at regular intervals.

Surgery should not be performed, if possible, until at least 6 weeks after this drug has been discontinued.

Hepatic tumours have occurred in some patients, some malignant others not.

The following conditions have been adversely affected by treatment: enlargement of uterine fibroids, exacerbation or development of diabetes mellitus, increase in blood pressure, the development of jaundice, amenorrhoea during and after therapy, depression, fluid retention and hence conditions such as epilepsy, migraine, asthma, cardiac and renal dysfunction, varicose veins, multiple sclerosis, the wearing of contact lenses and any condition which worsened during pregnancy.

Breakthrough bleeding may occur which manifests as bleeding outside the usual period.

Effects:
Central nervous system: headaches, exacerbation of migraine and epilepsy.

Gastrointestinal: nausea, vomiting, change in weight.

Genitourinary: breakthrough bleeding, spotting, irregular menstrual pattern.

Breast changes.

Skin: pigmentation.

CHEM NAME	TRADE NAME	FORMULATION
dydrogesterone	DUPHASTON	10mg

Dysmenorrhoea: 1 twice daily from day 5 to day 25 of the cycle.
Endometriosis: 1 twice or three times daily from day 5 to day 25 of the cycle or continuously.
Premenstrual syndrome: 1 twice daily from day 12 to day 26 of the cycle.
Hormone replacement therapy: 2 daily for 12 days each month.

medroxy-progesterone	PROVERA	5mg

2.5–10mg daily for five to ten days. Repeat on two to three consecutive cycles.

norethisterone	MENZOL	5mg
	PRIMOLUT N	5mg
	UTOVLAN	5mg

Postponement of menses: 1 three times daily starting three days before the expected onset of the menses.
Dysmenorrhoea: 1 three times daily from day 5 to day 25 of the cycle then none. Maintain for three to four cycles.
Menorrhagia/Premenstrual syndrome: 1 twice or three times daily from day 19 to day 26 of the cycle.

| progesterone | CYCLOGEST | 200mg, 400mg suppositories |

200–400mg rectally or vaginally once or twice daily from day 12 or 14 of the cycle until the menses commence.

Anabolic Steroids and Androgens

Androgens are hormones which lead to the development of secondary sexual characteristics in men. They are not commonly used. They may be prescribed to stimulate appetite, increase weight, help convalscence from illness.

The details below refer to them as a group. The classical male hormone, testosterone, has the most effect on male secondary sexual characteristics. It should however be borne in mind that the others also have masculinising effects even in low doses and so this effect is especially noted in those before puberty and in females.

Contraindications:
Known or suspected prostatic or breast cancer, high serum calcium levels, nephrotic syndrome, ischaemic heart disease or untreated cardiac failure.

Precautions:
Care must be exercised in the elderly, those with cardiac failure, renal or liver disease, hypertension, epilepsy and migraine. A history of these conditions should also lead to careful monitoring.

Effects:
General: hoarse voice, other signs of virilisation such as growth of facial hair and temporal recession of hair. The voice changes are initially temporary and then become permanent.
Cardiovascular: oedema, high blood pressure.

Respiratory: polyps of larynx.

Gastrointestinal: (these depend upon the exact chemical given) jaundice, liver tumours — benign and malignant.

Psychological: confusional state.

Urogenital: priapism, excessive sexual stimulation, precocious sexual development, increased frequency of erections, phallic enlargement in pre-pubertal males, decreased sperm count, menstrual irregularities.

Skin: acne, hirsutism.

CHEM NAME	TRADE NAME	FORMULATION
mesterolone	PRO-VIRON	25mg

Maintenance 2–3 daily.

stanozolol	STROMBA	5mg

Variable dose. 10mg daily is a fairly high dose.
This is the classical anabolic steroid and is one of the substances which all the fuss is about with regard to building muscle bulk among sportsmen and athletes. It is used medically in general practice for people who are underweight. An invidious practice to say the least. It underlines the remarkable lack of understanding of the origin of imbalances.

testosterone	RESTANDOL	40mg

1–3 daily.

Oral Contraceptives

The details here should be compared with the details of an oestrogen and a progestogen separately as above. I have listed these in detail not to repeat this information but because the dosages given in the form of contraception are lower. Therefore, when looking at side-effects particularly I would refer you to the section on page 262.

Contraindications:

Existing thrombophlebitis, thrombosis, cerebral vascular disease, myocardial infarction or a past history of these conditions. Also excluded are patients with sickle-cell anaemia, impaired liver function, disorders of lipid metabolism, known or suspected carcinoma of the breast, known or suspected oestrogen-dependent tumours, history during pregnancy of jaundice, itching, shingles or deterioration of otosclerosis, undiagnosed abnormal genital tract bleeding and known or suspected pregnancy.

Warnings:

There is an increased risk of thrombophlebitis, cerebrovascular disorders, myocardial infarction and pulmonary embolism. Some cases have proved fatal. This risk is increased in the presence of smoking, obesity, varicose veins, cardiovascular disease, diabetes mellitus and migraine and as age increases.

Surgery should not be performed, if possible, for at least 6 weeks after the drug has been stopped.

There is an increased incidence of gall bladder disease in patients who take these compounds.

Some patients have developed liver tumours, some malignant others not.

Precautions:

Certain conditions may be affected by this drug:

Uterine fibroids increase in size, diabetes mellitus exacerbated or precipitated, increase in blood pressure, the appearance of jaundice, amenorrhoea during or after therapy, depression, fluid retention and hence the exacerbation of epilepsy, migraine, asthma, cardiac and renal dysfunction, varicose veins, multiple sclerosis, the wearing of contact lenses or any condition which worsened during pregnancy.

Effects:

General: fatigue, Vitamin B6 deficiency.

Cardiovascular: oedema, hypertension, thromboembolism, peripheral ischaemia (this has resulted in some cases of amputation). Raised cholesterol levels.

Respiratory: increased number of respiratory infections, nasal catarrh, allergic rhinitis.

Central nervous system: headache, migraine. EEG changes are seen in up to 60% of women who take the combined oral contraceptive.

Psychological: premenstrual-like syndrome, changes in libido, nervousness, depression.

Gastrointestinal: gum hypertrophy, nausea, vomiting, diarrhoea, abdominal pain, pancreatitis, Crohn's disease, change in weight, effects on vitamin and mineral levels. Liver function test changes, increased incidence of gall bladder disease.

Genitourinary: breakthrough bleeding, spotting, change in menstrual flow, amenorrhoea, cervical erosions and secretions, vaginal thrush, cystitis-like syndrome, increased number of urinary tract infections.

Breast changes: enlargement, tenderness, secretion, suppression of lactation.

Musculosceletal: inflammation of tendons and joints

Skin: rashes, pigmentation, hirsutism, loss of scalp hair, itching, acne, Candida infections ('thrush'), urticaria, eczema.
Special senses: worsening of otosclerosis, intolerance to contact lenses.
The combined contraceptive pills often contain varying relative amounts of oestrogen and progesterone over the month. I have omitted the exact details.

Combined Pill (Oestrogen and Progesterone)

CHEM NAME	TRADE NAME	FORMULATION
ethinyl-oestradiol	BINOVUM	with norethisterone
	BREVINOR	with norethisterone
	CONOVA 30	with ethynodiol
	EUGYNON 30	with norgestrel
	FEMODENE	with gestodene
	FEMODENE ED	with gestodene
	LOESTRIN 20	with norethisterone
	LOESTRIN 30	with norethisterone
	LOGYNON	with levonorgestrel
	LOGYNON ED	with levonorgestrel
	MARVELON	with desogestrel
	MERCILON	with desogestrel
	MICROGYNON 30	with levonorgestrel
	MINULET	with gestodene
	NEOCON 1/35	with norethisterone
	NORIMIN	with norethisterone
	OVRAN	with levonorgestrel
	OVRAN 30	with levonorgestrel
	OVRANETTE	with levonorgestrel
	OVYSMEN	with norethisterone
	SYNPHASE	with 5mg norethisterone
	TRINORDIOL	with levonorgestrel
	TRINOVUM	with norethisterone
	TRINOVUM ED	with norethisterone
mestranol	NORINYL-1	50mcg with 1mg norethisterone
	ORTHO-NOVIN 1/50	50mcg with 1mg norethisterone

In general, these are taken for 21 days in sequence then 7 tablet free days during which time bleeding will occur. I am reluctant to call this menstruation since it only occurs due to a withdrawal of the medication for this time. Therefore, it should be known as 'withdrawal bleeding'.

Minipill (Progestogen Only)

For details of contraindications, precautions and effects see the entry under progesterone on page 266.

CHEM NAME	TRADE NAME	FORMULATION
ethynodiol	FEMULEN	500mcg
One daily starting on the first day of menstruation and taken without a break.		
levonorgestrel	MICROVAL	30mcg
	NORGESTON	30mcg
One daily starting on the first day of menstruation and taken without a break.		
norethisterone	MICRONOR	350mcg
	NORIDAY	350mcg
One daily starting on the first day of menstruation and taken without a break.		
norgestrel	NEOGEST	75mcg
One daily starting on the first day of menstruation and taken without a break.		

COMMENTS

I will discuss all sex hormones together as they are similar compounds and it is mainly variation in dose which differentiates hormone replacement therapy in the menopause (HRT) from oral contraception, for example.

Oestrogens and progestogens are given either alone or in combination and are the hormones normally produced by the ovary during the menstrual cycle.

They are widely used for contraception, HRT and menstrual disorders. There is a current epidemic of prescriptions for use in menopausal and post-menopausal women for the treatment of symptoms of flushing, emotional instability and other results of 'oestrogen deficiency' as well as to reputedly prevent the later development of osteoporosis. I shall take the conventional view first to discuss the pros and cons of hormone therapy.

Firstly, all these compounds have similar effects which reflect their relatedness. They lead to thrombosis, 'stroke', high blood pressure and will exacerbate hormone-dependent tumours of the breast and uterus. Oestrogens used alone are linked to the development of endometrial carcinoma — the addition of progestogens is reputed to remove this risk.

There is an on-going controversy regarding a connection between breast cancer and the oral contraceptive with recent studies revealing an alarming increase in the risk of cancer for women who take this drug.[13] It would seem to be clear to me that if a drug leads to the worsening of a condition it is also implicated in its development. Therefore, the oral contraceptive pill and HRT would seem to increase the risk of developing breast cancer. There may also be a connection between these compounds and abnormalities of the uterine cervix — these are increasing in number and found in ever younger women.

A similar controversy surrounds the use of HRT with studies which show a relationship between breast cancer and HRT criticised by the medical profession. The resultant view is that no-one knows but in the meantime HRT should be continued and indeed used in increasing numbers of women. I find this attitude surprising if not downright dangerous. If there is a risk of a serious disease such as breast cancer resulting from treatment with a certain drug it seems to be irresponsible to carry on as usual as if there were NO evidence. How much evidence is required? Meanwhile patients are the pawns in this game played out by doctors and the pharmaceutical industry.

There is however solid recent evidence that HRT definitely leads to the development of breast cancer with an increase in risk of 10% with treatment of more than 5 years.[14]

Apart from cancer development the numerous other side-effects are commonly seen in women who take these hormones — either mental, emotional or physical — and, indeed, a whole generation of women has grown up taking these chemicals for contraception.[15] It has taken 20–30 years for the conventional profession to even suspect these connections, I would expect a similar period of time to elapse before the dangers of HRT are realised.

HRT definitely relieves the symptoms associated with the menopause in most cases and patients feel very much better. Osteoporosis is a condition which occurs later in life and is by no means universal. If HRT is to be continued after the menopause to prevent this then it would seem sensible to ensure the following:

1. There should be no contraindications such as history of thrombosis, myocardial infarction, otosclerosis, known or suspected hormone-dependent cancer, undiagnosed abnormal genital bleeding.
2. Regular checks should be made of breast, pelvis (vaginal examination) and blood pressure with a pre-treatment check. Regular means annual.
3. Patients should be pre-selected so that those who are most likely to develop osteoporosis are treated, i.e. slightly built, thin and smokers.
4. Patients should be fully informed of the side-effects of treatment and its dangers especially with regard to breast cancer.
5. Oestrogens must never be prescribed alone to a women with a uterus because of the risk of endometrial cancer.

Now to discuss hormone treatment from a more alternative view-point. All these hormones are basically of the steroid type. There are a lot of similarities in actions. They would seem to be as suppressive in their own way.

The oral contraceptive, for example, stops menstruation and patients only bleed every month because the drugs are withheld for 7 days. The correct name for this event then is 'withdrawal bleeding' — not menstruation. This suppression of menstruation, as with the suppression of any discharge from the body is potentially harmful. The homoeopathic texts abound with remedies used for this guiding symptom.[16]

So it can be seen that the oral contraceptive pill will eventually erode the patient's health. Any treatment given while the patient takes these drugs will necessarily be limited in its effectiveness and I always discuss the subject of contraception to enable patients to consider alternatives.

In my experience every patient has been concerned about taking the oral contraceptive although those fears are often unvoiced. Also, most patients have considered other forms of contraception and stopped the 'pill' during treatment.

Energetically, these drugs not only 'stop' menstruation they stagnate the flow of energy generally and the conditions of pre-menstrual syndrome, breast tumours — benign and malignant — and uterine cervical abnormalities are the result of this stagnation. This relationship is clearly seen in Chinese Medicine and merely underlines the effect of these drugs.

Another problem with these drugs is the peculiar mental and emotional effects they produce. Some women become depressed or irritable and therefore stop the medication. Others become almost euphoric (compare with the mental effects of the corticosteroids which can develop into a 'steroid psychosis'). This euphoric state is noted for its lack of insight and treating patients who take HRT can be very difficult.

I call it the 'Dynasty' syndrome in that there is a false 'high' of youthful vigour, sexual attractiveness and general apparent lack of ageing. This, I guess, is the core of the issue. The alternative to HRT is ageing, the inevitable deterioration of the physical body. It is advertised as the drug which will prevent this.

Osteoporosis, actually, is not a disease but rather a natural concomitant of increasing age. It may be severe in some people due to life-style or constitutional factors but it cannot be prevented, only limited. The one factor definitely involved in its development is lack of activity. Even active people in Western society have much less activity than in our rural past and this leads to diminution in bone density.

Calcium supplementation is irrelevant[17] and has always been recognised as such although with reduction in milk quotas in the EC the Milk Marketing Board is looking for other avenues to use its products.

What to do with such cases?

These drugs, to summarise, lead to mental and emotional changes, a risk of breast cancer and uterine disease as well as various vascular conditions such as thrombosis and 'stroke'.

Alternative forms of contraception need to be discussed with the patient and her partner and made available

In the case of HRT, alternative medicine offers a viable source of relief of symptoms around the menopause and the nature of osteoporosis should be explained as well as actions the patient can take to minimise its harmful effects.

When actually treating patients who take HRT sudden withdrawal can lead to marked feelings of ill-health, depression and tiredness. There may also be menstrual irregularities in patients who still have that potential.

Gradual reduction is therefore helpful if possible and this is somewhat dependent on the formulation administered. Surgical implants last for 6 months or so but there are a variety of dosages which can be used. Patches or plasters can be used less frequently and the same with tablets.

Problems may ensue in women who still have a uterus.

Bleeding may occur at irregular intervals as the dose is reduced so here it is necessary to stop the drug and treat as required. This is to avoid a situation where the patient experiences a lot of spotting or breakthrough bleeding whilst the dosage is reduced.

The main hurdle is acceptance by the patient of her natural process. There may be resistance from family or partner to seeing her grow old. Menopause is not a disease — it is a normal stage of development just as birth, puberty and death. HRT is the direct result of Western society's false view of reality which sees events and people as static and unchanging. This is the area where the therapist can help the patient learn a new way of being.

13 DERMATOLOGY

CORTICOSTEROIDS FOR THE SKIN

Applications may be in several forms according to the condition or its presentation. Creams, ointments and lotions are available in most cases. It is the strength which is the important factor eg 1%, 0.5% and so on. Even if there is no milder strength the pharmacist can produce one by dilution with a plain moisturising cream.

Contraindications:

Rosacea, acne vulgaris and peri-oral dermatitis or with primary viral infections of the skin such as herpes simplex or chickenpox. It should also not be used in infected skin lesions or for children under 1 year of age.

Precautions:

Long-term treatment should be avoided wherever possible especially in infants and children. This is because of adrenal suppression.

The face especially, and other areas of the body, may suffer atrophic changes in the skin after prolonged treatment.

In childhood or in cases of facial skin disease, courses of treatment should be kept to 5 days and occlusion not used.

These agents may be hazardous in psoriasis due to the development of tolerance, worsening of the disease on withdrawal and the development of toxic effects.

Effects:

As with systemic corticosteroids there is a danger of masking or aggravation of an underlying infection.

The severity and frequency of these depend on the actual potency of the steroid used.

Skin: local effects include dermatitis, acne, worsening of rosacea, wrinkling of skin, thinning of skin, striae, dilatation of blood vessels, susceptible to injury, delay in wound healing, worsening of ulceration, hypo- and hyperpigmentation. Urticaria. Photosensitivity. These local effects are exaggerated by the use of occlusive dressings.

Prolonged use may suppress adrenal function especially in children and babies.

Psoriasis may develop into the pustular form of the disease when treated with corticosteroids.

MILDLY POTENT CORTICOSTEROID

CHEM NAME	TRADE NAME	FORMULATION
alcomethasone	MODRASONE	0.05%
fluocinolone	SYNALAR 1:10	0.0025%
hydrocortisone	ACTINAC	1% with chloramphenicol, butoxyethyl,
base or acetate		allantoin and sulphur

With the addition of an antibacterial and a keratolytic.
Used in the treatment of acne.

	ALPHOSYL HC	0.5% with coal tar, allantoin

With the addition of an antipsoriatic.
Used in the treatment of psoriasis.

	BARQUINOL HC	0.5% with clioquinol

With the addition of an antibacterial/antifungal.

	CANESTEN HC	1% with clotrimazole

With the addition of an antifungal.

	CARBOCORT	0.25% with coal tar

With the addition of an antipsoriatic.

	COBADEX	0.5%, 1% with dimethicone

With the addition of a barrier agent.

	DAKTACORT	1% with miconazole 2%

With the addition of an antifungal.

	DIODERM	0.1%
	ECONACORT	1% with econazole

With the addition of an antifungal.

	ECZEDERM-HC	0.5% with calamine, arachis oil

With the addition of an anti-itching agent and an emollient.

	EFCORTELAN	0.5%, 1% 2.5%
	EPIFOAM	1% with pramoxine

With the addition of a local anaesthetic.

	EURAX- Hydrocortisone	0.25% with crotamiton

With the addition of an anti-itching agent.

	FRAMYCORT	0.5% with framycetin

With the addition of an antibacterial.

	FUCIDIN H	1% with sodium fusidate

With the addition of an antibacterial.

GENTICIN HC 1% with gentamicin
With the addition of an antibacterial.

GREGODERM 1% with neomycin,
nystatin, polymyxin B
With the addition of an antibacterial and antifungals.

HYDROCAL 1% with calamine
With the addition of an anti-itching agent.

HYDROCORTISTAB 1%
HYDROCORTISYL 1%
MILDISON 1%
LIPOCREAM
NYSTAFORM HC 0.5% with nystatin,
chlorhexidine
With the addition of an antifungal and an antibacterial.

QUINOCORT 1% with potassium
hydroxyquinoline
sulphate
With the addition of an antibacterial/antifungal.

QUINODERM with 1% with benzoyl
HYDRO peroxide, potassium
-CORTISONE hydroxyquinoline
sulphate
With the addition of an antibacterial and a keratolytic.
Used in the treatment of acne.

SENTIAL 0.5% with urea, sodium
chloride
With the addition of an hydrating agent.

TARCORTIN 0.5% with coal tar
With the addition of an antipsoriatic.

TERRA-CORTRIL 1% with oxytetracycline
With the addition of an antibacterial.

TERRA-CORTRIL 1% with oxytetracycline,
NYSTATIN nystatin
With the addition of an antibacterial and an antifungal.

TIMODINE 0.5% with nystatin,
benzalkonium,
dimethicone
With the addition of an antifungal, antibacterial and a disinfectant.

TRICICATRIN 1% with neomycin,
bacitracin, nystatin
With the addition of antibacterials and an antifungal.

VIOFORM- 1% with clioquinol
Hydrocortisone
With the addition of an antibacterial/antifungal.

| methyl-prednisolone | MEDRONE | 0.25% with sulphur, aluminium chlorhydroxide |

With the addition of a keratolytic.
Used in the treatment of acne.

| | NEO-MEDRONE | 0.25% with neomycin |

With the addition of an antibacterial.

MODERATELY POTENT CORTICOSTEROID

CHEM NAME	TRADE NAME	FORMULATION
clobetasone	EUMOVATE	0.05%
	TRIMOVATE	0.05% with nystatin, tetracycline

With the addition of an antifungal and an antibacterial.

| desoxymethasone | STIEDEX LP | 0.05% |
| | STIEDEX LP N | 0.05% with neomycin |

With the addition of an antibacterial.

fluocinolone	SYNALAR 1:4	0.00625%
fluocortolone	ULTRADIL	0.1%
	ULTRALANUM	0.25%
flurandrenolone	HAELAN	0.0125%
	HAELAN TAPE	in unresponsive conditions
	HAELAN-X	0.05%
	HAELAN-C	0.0125% with clioquinol

With the addition of an antifungal/antibacterial.

| hydrocortisone | ALPHADERM | 1% with urea |

With the addition of an hydrating agent.

| | CALMURID HC | 1% with urea, lactic acid |

With the addition of an hydrating agent and a keratolytic.

POTENT CORTICOSTEROID

CHEM NAME	TRADE NAME	FORMULATION
beclomethasone	PROPADERM	0.025%
	PROPADERM A	0.025% with chlortetracycline

With the addition of an antibacterial.

| betamethasone | BETNOVATE | 0.1%, scalp application |

		0.1%
	BETNOVATE C	0.1% with clioquinol

With the addition of an antifungal/antibacterial.

	BETNOVATE N	0.1% with neomycin

With the addition of an antibacterial.

	BETNOVATE RD	0.025%
	DIPROSALIC	0.05%, scalp application 0.05% both with salicylic acid

With the addition of a keratolytic.

	DIPROSONE	0.05%, lotion 0.05%
	FUCIBET	0.1% with fusidic acid

With the addition of an antibacterial.

	LOTRIDERM	0.05% with clotrimazole

With the addition of an antibacterial/antifungal.

budesonide	PREFERID	0.025%
desoxymethasone	STIEDEX	0.25%
diflucortolone	NERISONE	0.1%
fluclorolone	TOPILAR	0.025%
fluocinolone	SYNALAR	0.025%
	SYNALAR GEL	0.025% for scalp
	SYNALAR C	0.025% with clioquinol

With the addition of an antifungal/antibacterial.

	SYNALAR N	0.025% with neomycin

With the addition of an antibacterial.

fluocinonide	METOSYN	0.05%, scalp application 0.05%
hydrocortisone 17-butyrate	LOCOID	0.1%, scalp application 0.1%
	LOCOID C	with chlorquinaldol

With the addition of an antifungal/antibacterial.

triamcinolone	ADCORTYL	0.1%
	ADCORTYL with GRANEODIN	0.1% with neomycin, gramicidin

With the addition of antibacterials.

	AUREOCORT	0.1% with chlortetracycline

With the addition of an antibacterial.

	LEDERCORT	0.1%
	NYSTADERMAL	0.1% with nystatin

With the addition of an antifungal.

	PEVARYL TC	0.1% with econazole

With the addition of an antifungal.

	TRI-ADCORTYL	0.1% with nystatin,

neomycin, gramicidin
With the addition of an antifungal and antibacterials.

VERY POTENT CORTICOSTEROID

CHEM NAME	TRADE NAME	FORMULATION
clobetasol	DERMOVATE	0.05%, scalp application 0.05%
	DERMOVATE NN	0.05% with neomycin, nystatin

With the addition of an antifungal and an antibacterial.

diflucortolone	NERISONE FORTE	0.3%
halcinonide	HALCIDERM	0.1%

COMMENTS

All the above applications should be considered to be in Category III as outlined on page 18. Slow withdrawal is essential because of the danger of the release of suppressed symptoms.

Topical corticosteroids are used for a wide variety of skin disorders such as eczema, psoriasis and dermatitis where suppression of inflammation is required. They are also used with antibiotics or antifungal agents where infection is present. Whilst the correct conventional approach is to use the mildest product possible they are widely available and prescribed. The mild applications can harm the structure of the skin in the long term. Mild hydrocortisone creams are also available over-the-counter. The addition of antibacterial and antifungal agents to creams is associated with a high risk of allergic responses.

This suppressive action can lead to the development of severe internal disease as the skin rash disappears.[18] Treatment leads to the release of suppression so that the rash may increase in the short-term and removal of the steroid applications may also do the same. Slow reduction of the dosage whilst treatment is progressing will minimise the risk of an exacerbation of the symptoms which is difficult to deal with. This is especially true for facial problems where patients are very reluctant to tolerate a worsening of the skin symptoms.

The prescription of progressively weaker applications can also be helpful in gradually reducing the dose of steroid put on the skin.

The effects of all the steroid applications are similar although the weaker applications will tend to be less severe and for the very potent applications more so.

Skin Preparations

These are used to relieve symptoms due to dryness, scaling and for itching. They are used when necessary and may be given as creams, ointments or lotions.

ANTI-ITCHING AGENTS

CHEM NAME	TRADE NAME	FORMULATION
calamine	CALADRYL	with camphor, diphenhydramine
With the addition of an antihistamine.		
	ECZEDERM	with arachis oil
With the addition of an emollient.		
	R.B.C.	with antazoline, camphor, cetrimide
With the addition of an antihistamine and an antibacterial.		
crotamiton	EURAX	

ANTISEPTIC

CHEM NAME	TRADE NAME	FORMULATION
calendula	CALENDOLON	

SKIN PROTECTANT

CHEM NAME	TRADE NAME	FORMULATION
carmellose	ORABASE ORAHESIVE	

EMOLLIENT

CHEM NAME	TRADE NAME	FORMULATION
chamomile oil	KAMILLOSAN	
cod liver oil	MORHULIN	with zinc oxide
liquid paraffin	ALCODERM	
	ALPHA KERI	
	KERI	
	DIPROBASE	with soft paraffin
	E45	with soft paraffin
	EMULSIDERM	with benzalkonium

With the addition of an antibacterial.

	HYDROMOL	
	LIPOBASE	with soft paraffin
	LOCOBASE	
	OILATUM EMOLLIENT	with wool alcohols
	ULTRABASE	with soft paraffin
	UNGUENTUM	with soft paraffin, silicic acid, glycerol

With the addition of a keratolytic.

vitamin A	MORSEP	with cetrimide palmitate

With the addition of an antiseptic.

oat fraction	AVEENO	Regular
	AVEENO OILATED	with liquid paraffin
sodium pyrrolidone	HUMIDERM	
	LACTICARE	with lactic acid

With the addition of a keratolytic.

soya oil	BALNEUM	

For use in bath.

squalane	DERMALEX	with hexachlorophane, allantoin

With the addition of an antiseptic.

	NATUDERM	with glycerides, glycerol
urea	AQUADRATE	
	NUTRAPLUS	
	CALMURID	with lactic acid

With the addition of a keratolytic.

	SENTIAL E	with sodium chloride
wool fat	SUDOCREM	with zinc oxide, benzyl benzoate

With the addition of an antiseptic.

	THOVALINE	with zinc oxide, talc, kaolin, cod liver oil

With the addition of an antiseptic.

LOCAL ANAESTHETIC

CHEM NAME	TRADE NAME	FORMULATION
cinchocaine	NUPERCAINAL	

FATTY ACID

CHEM NAME	TRADE NAME	FORMULATION
gamolenic acid	EPOGAM	40mg

4–6 twice daily.
Children: under 1 year not recommended, over 1 year 2–4 twice daily.
Used to treat eczema.

ANTISEPTIC

CHEM NAME	TRADE NAME	FORMULATION
sodium chloride	MIOL	with magnesium chloride and others

Mixture of antiseptic agents.

COMMENTS

Some of these preparations are fairly innocuous and there is no harm in using simple moisturisers (emollients) for dry skin conditions and eczema. Problems may begin when applications contain other compounds such as an anti-itching agent or an antihistamine.

Substances made from either petroleum (liquid paraffin and soft paraffin) or wool fat (lanolin) may be responsible for allergic reactions. These reactions may be indistinguishable from the original condition.

Psoriasis

Many of these are non-specific agents to help with problems of scaling of skin. Others are specific drugs aimed to counteract the excessive growth of skin cells — a characteristic feature of psoriasis.

ANTIBACTERIAL

CHEM NAME	TRADE NAME	FORMULATION
benzalkonium Shampoo.	CAPITOL	gel

ANTISEPTIC

CHEM NAME	TRADE NAME	FORMULATION
cetrimide Shampoo.	CEANEL Conc.	with alcohol

ANTIPSORIATIC

CHEM NAME	TRADE NAME	FORMULATION
coal tar	ALPHOSYL	with allantoin
	BALNEUM with TAR	with soya oil
With the addition of an emollient.		
	BALTAR	
Shampoo.		
	CARBO-DOME	
	CLINITAR	
	GELCOSAL	with tar, salicylic acid
With the addition of a keratolytic.		
	GELCOTAR	with tar
	GENISOL	liquid
Shampoo.		
	IONIL T	with benzalkonium,

		salicylic acid

With the addition of a keratolytic.

	POLYTAR EMOLLIENT	with arachis oil
	POLYTAR Liquid	with arachis oil

Shampoo.
BWith the addition of an emollient.

	POLYTAR PLUS	with arachis oil (contains animal protein)

Shampoo.

	PRAGMATAR	with sulphur, salicylic acid
	PSORIDERM	
	PSORIGEL	
	PSORIN	with dithranol, salicylic acid

With the addition of a keratolytic.

	T GEL	

Shampoo.

dithranol	ANTHRANOL	0.4%, 1%, 2%
	ANTRADERM	1%
	ANTRADERM MILD	0.5%
	ANTRADERM FORTE	2%
	DITHROCREAM	0.1%, 0.25%
	DITHROCREAM FORTE	0.5%
	DITHROCREAM HP	1%
	DITHROCREAM 2%	2%
	DITHROLAN	0.5% with salicylic acid

With the addition of a keratolytic.

	EXOLAN	1% cream
	PSORADRATE	0.1%, 0.2% or 0.4% all with urea

With the addition of an emollient.

FUNGICIDE/BACTERICIDE

CHEM NAME	TRADE NAME	FORMULATION
mono-alkylolamide Shampoo.	SYNOGIST	

ANTISEPTIC

CHEM NAME	TRADE NAME	FORMULATION
cetrimide	CRADOCAP	10%
For cradle cap in children.		
povidone-iodine	BETADINE	

ANTIDANDRUFF AGENT

CHEM NAME	TRADE NAME	FORMULATION
selenium	LENIUM	
	SELSUN	
Shampoo.		

COMMENTS

Applications used in the treatment of psoriasis (as those used for eczema) may well contain substances which are suppressive and harmful. Sulphur has been known for centuries to remove the symptoms of skin disease. However, given in large quantities as here, it can only be suppressive in action. Sulphur as used by homoeopaths is a completely different situation.

Tar based compounds and its synthetic derivative, dithranol, lead to relief of symptoms but suppression of the problem leading either to more resistant skin problems or to internal disease at some date in the future.

The use of corticosteroid creams in the treatment of psoriasis makes the condition worse in the long-term although short-term symptomatic relief is obtained. This is recognised conventionally.[19]

Treatment of patients can be very difficult since they come for consultation when the rash is fairly mild and yet there may be a vast amount of suppressed material which can reappear when treatment begins and/or when the application is reduced or withdrawn.

A last point about treating skin conditions. On occasion it can be very difficult to deal with the feelings expressed towards you as a result of the natural healing process. It may be preferable to ask patients to gradually reduce their medication and return later. In this way you see the skin problem in its natural form and you would not be held responsible for any worsening as the drug is withdrawn.

Acne

ABRASIVE

CHEM NAME	TRADE NAME	FORMULATION
aluminium oxide	BRASIVOL	abrasive paste (fine, medium, coarse)
polyethylene granules	IONAX	with benzalkonium
With the addition of an antibacterial.		

ANTIBACTERIAL/KERATOLYTIC

CHEM NAME	TRADE NAME	FORMULATION
benzalkonium	TORBETOL	with cetrimide, hexachlorophane
With the addition of other antibacterials.		
benzoyl peroxide	ACETOXYL	2.5%, 5%
	ACNEGEL	5%
	ACNEGEL FORTE	10%
	ACNIDAZIL	5% with miconazole
With the addition of an antifungal.		
	BENZOYL 5	5%
	BENZOYL 5 SULPHUR	with 5% with sulphur
	BENZOYL 10	10%
	BENZOYL 10 SULPHUR	with 10% with sulphur
	BENZAGEL	5%, 10%
	NERICUR	5%, 10%
	PANOXYL	5%, 10%
	PANOXYL AQUAGEL	2.5%, 5%, 10%
	PANOXYL WASH	10%
	QUINODERM	10% with potassium

With the addition of a keratolytic.

	hydroxyquinoline sulphate
QUINODERM CREAM 5	5% with potassium hydroxyquinoline sulphate

With the addition of a keratolytic.

QUINODERM LOTIO-GEL	10% with potassium hydroxyquinoline sulphate

With the addition of a keratolytic.

QUINODERM LOTIO-GEL	5% with potassium hydroxyquinoline sulphate 5%

With the addition of a keratolytic.

ANTIBIOTIC

CHEM NAME	TRADE NAME	FORMULATION
clindamycin	DALACIN T	
erythromycin	STIEMYCIN	
	ZINERYT	
tetracycline	TOPICYCLINE	

These are all in the form of solutions for local use. Oral antibiotics particularly the tetracyclines and erythromycin may be given long-term.

ANTI-ANDROGEN
Effects:
General: tiredness, drowsiness, weakness.
Gastrointestinal: weight change, decreased glucose tolerance in diabetics.
Psychological: depression.
Endocrine: breast pain and tenderness (10%), breast enlargement, galactorrhoea.
Urogenital: genital pain.
Skin: decreased body hair.

CHEM NAME	TRADE NAME	FORMULATION
cyproterone	DIANETTE	2mg with 35mcg ethinyloestradiol

1 daily for 21 days then 7 tablet free days (menstruation should occur during this time).
With the addition of an oestrogen. Only for females. The same comments made under the oral contraceptives are valid here.
Cyproterone is a steroid base and leads to amenorrhoea and irregular uterine bleeding. Therefore it is combined with an oestrogen and given on a cyclical basis.
The oral contraceptive pill may be given to some females with acne.

KERATOLYTIC

CHEM NAME	TRADE NAME	FORMULATION
resorcinol	ESKAMEL	2% with sulphur

VITAMIN A DERIVATIVE

This is a powerful drug and has many effects.
General: tiredness, fatigue, sleepiness, lethargy, musculoskele-tal pain.
Gastrointestinal: angular stomatitis, gingivitis, glossitis, anorexia, nausea, vomiting, weight loss, epigastric pain, thirst, spleen and liver enlargement, liver function test changes.
Central nervous system: vertigo.
Psychological: irritability, sleep disturbances, psychological changes.
Urogenital: increased menstrual bleeding,
Skin: these reactions occur in up to 70% of patients. Scaling of skin, dry mucous membranes, erythema, itching, disturbed hair growth, thinning of hair.
Special senses: epistaxis, double vision, conjunctivitis.

CHEM NAME	TRADE NAME	FORMULATION
tretinoin	RETIN-A	0.025%
	RETIN-A CREAM	0.025%, 0.05%

COMMENTS

Again, there is no harm in using a skin cleanser which does not contain chemicals (there are few here I may add) which will lead to a reduction in oiliness and so less blocked pores. The use of antibiotics, hormones and the like can only suppress and not cure. Treatment is difficult because the real picture of the skin condition is hidden by the drugs. Only when they are withdrawn does this become evident.

Table of drugs used in increasing order of severity:

- cleansers, abrasives, keratolytics
- antibiotic — local
- antibiotic — oral
- Vitamin A derivative
- antiandrogen
- oral contraceptive

It is possible to treat at the same time as reduction in dosage takes place but as with psoriasis and other skin conditions the therapist may be held responsible for the worsening condition of the face. This, in a teenager, may be too much for the patient to bear.

It is essential that the therapist approaches this situation with care. It is preferable, and certainly possible in most cases, to ask the patient to stop the medication over the period of a month or so and then to return for treatment. In such a way it is possible to see the real clinical picture, the drugs will not interfere with the treatment and the therapist will not be accused of being responsible for the appearance of spots on the patient's face.

14   END-NOTES

SYMPTOMATIC DRUGS

The easiest situation to deal with is someone who is taking drugs purely for symptomatic relief. This is category I as outlined on page 18. If a patient takes, for example, analgesics or laxatives for the relief of a symptom, they usually only do so when that symptom appears.

There will few problems with treatment and as the condition improves the drugs will no longer be needed.

However, if the drugs are taken every day then it becomes more of a long term problem, more like category IV as before and so is more difficult.

The drugs considered to be symptomatic are those taken infrequently for a symptom:

- analgesics
- cough medicines
- laxatives
- nasal sprays
- antacids

They are all fairly mild, will not interfere unduly with treatment and do not mask the picture of the symptoms.

FOOT-NOTES

1. Throughout this book the emphasis is on treatment by alternative medicine and this is implied whenever management or treatment is mentioned. When reference is made to conventional medicine this is clearly distinguished.

   Some 18% of men and 25% of women in the U.K. regularly take prescription medication. When this is added to those taking over-the-counter remedies there are clearly large sections of the population taking drugs for medical conditions.
2. Medicines: A Guide for Everybody. Parrish (Allen Lane).
3. Organon of Medicine. S.Hahnemann (Gollancz) — Aphorism 37.
4. Health Shock. Martin Weitz (Hamlyn).
5. Concise Medical Dictionary (Oxford Medical Publications).
6. Cured to Death. Melville and Johnson (New English Library).
7. Health Shock. Martin Weitz (Hamlyn).
8. Davidson's Principles and Practice of Medicine. Edited by Macleod (Churchill Livingstone).
9. Lancet April 29th 1989.
10. MIMS Magazine May 1st 1989. 'Kidney Disorders in General Practice.'
11. Davidson's Principles and Practice of Medicine. Edited by Macleod (Churchill Livingstone).
12. Drugs and Therapeutics Bulletin Vol.27 No.8 April 1989.
13. Lancet May 6th 1989.
14. New England Journal of Medicine August 1989.
15. In 1979 some 40% of sexually active women between the age of 15 and 44 were using the oral contraceptive. (Family Planning Association).
16. Repertory of the Homoeopathic Materia Medica. Kent (World Homoeopathic Links).
17. MIMS Magazine December 1988.
18. The Chronic Diseases. S.Hahnemann (Jain).
19. Medical Monitor May 1989.

BIBLIOGRAPHY

ABPI Data Sheet Compendium. A basic source of information for the medical profession (provided by the pharmaceutical industry) giving details of drugs and their side-effects. A useful guide so long as it is not seen as the final word.

British National Formulary. Published several times a year and in terms of detail falls somewhere between the two above. Gives a reasonable conventional view of drug usage without the exceses of some general and hospital practice.

Chronic Diseases, Samuel Hahnemann. Although written some 150 years ago it is still relevant today revealing the results of suppressive treatment by conventional means. Describes several case studies illustrating this.

Cured to Death, Arabella Melville and Colin Johnson. Similar to *Health Shock* but takes a closer at drug treatment and the pharmaceutical industry. Rather more genteel than *Health Shock*!

Health Shock, Martin Weitz. An excellent book describing the problems of conventional treatment. Many references are listed and a good source of hard information. This does not pull any punches.

The Extra Pharmacopoiea 1982 (28th Edition), Martindale. This heavy textbook (weight and content) contains many details of drugs, their formulations, effects and so on.

Meyler's Side Effects of Drugs, edited by M.N.G.Dukes (10th Edition). Possibly the definitive book on side effects and uses of drugs. It contains many references to original papers and journals of occurrences of problems with drugs.

MIMS (Monthly Index of Medical Specialities). A monthly index of drugs. Not much more than a recipe book.

Science of Homoeopathy, George Vithoulkas. An excellent introduction to energetic medicine which should be required reading for all practitioners. Understanding these concepts leads to much clearer ideas about disease, its origins, development and how to relieve it.

Textbood of Adverse Drug Reactions, edited by D.M.Davies (3rd Edition). Similar to Meyler's but with less detail.

APPENDIX

It is not easy communicating with practitioners you have never met and this is particularly true of orthodox practitioners. As I have mentioned before it is probably preferable to develop systems of support including conventional help which are as open as possible. However if you do want to or need to write to a GP then the format below is the one to follow.

I always say to practitioners that they are consultants in health care. The patient has consulted you about their problem and so in the hierarchy of medical politics you are on an equal level to medical practitioners. Of course they will have more expertise in certain areas and you will have more expertise in others. Nevertheless the result is that you are professional colleagues.

The general tone of the letter should be polite yet firm. There is no point in being defensive or vague and at the same time do not expect difficulties. Simply state what you do, what you expect to happen and what you want to happen. You will probably have a specific request maybe to do with monitoring, drug interactions or help with drug withdrawals. Give an outline of the case and state your position. GP's will respond more positively if you present yourself in a positive, polite yet professional way.

Always type your letters on professional-looking notepaper and include your qualifications. If you have not contacted this particular GP before perhaps you would give a brief description of what you do and include a leaflet about your therapy. End your letter with an invitation to discuss this matter further should the GP wish it.

Sample Letter 1

The Clinic
Street
Town
County

Dr A.N.Other
78 Conventional Street
Hampstead
London

15.7.91.

Dear Dr Other,

Re: Mrs A. Choice, 14 Kington Boulevard, Richmond.

This woman recently came to see me for acupuncture treatment of her migraine and to help reduce her medication.

Her current medication is:
1. Inderal 40mg three times daily.
2. Paracetamol 500mg two four times daily.
3. Valium 5mg three times daily.

This is the type of problem which often responds to acupuncture treatment. I would envisage that she would gain relief from her headaches after a course of treatment. However, there may be more difficulty managing her medications. Her underlying problem seems to be one of anxiety and, again, acupuncture can help this as well as supporting her while reducing her tranquillisers. This tends to be a more long-term problem and she may well need help from other sources such as a counselling or a self-help group.

I would appreciate your help with reduction of her medication once she begins to improve.

I shall keep in touch about her progress. If you would like to discuss this further I can be contacted at the above address.

Yours sincerely,

Dr S Gascoigne MB.,ChB.,C.Ac.

GENERAL INDEX
(including disease names)

acne 33, 262, **289–292**
addiction 13
Addison's disease **62**
adrenal cortex insufficiency 20, 31, **62**
allergic disease **151–6**, 176, 285
anaemia **196–7**
anal fissure 205
analgesic nephropathy 210, 221, 242
anaphylaxis 151
(also see allergic disease)
angina pectoris 99, 112
ankylosing spondylitis 248
anxiety **77–90**, 99, 167
arrhythmia 20, 31, **55**, 133
arthritis 210, **242–257**
asthma 19, 27, 62, 100, 132, 148, 149,
    151, 156, 162, 164, 165, **166–179**, 181,
    189, 228, 259, 262
autoimmune disease 258

behavioural disorders 156
bronchitis 151

cancer 274 bowel 202 breast 273, 275
    stomach 195 uterus (endometrium)
    273, 274
(also see tumours)
candidiasis 48, 150
cardiac arrhythmia (see arrhythmia)
cardiac failure 106, 109, 110, 118, 125,
    129, **130–4**
cervical dysplasia 273
Chinese medicine 17
chronic bronchitis 100, 166
colitis **205–9**
(also see ulcerative colitis)
conflict 15
constipation 184, 196, **197–202**
contraception 262, **269–272**
continuous release 21
contraindications 22
coronary thrombosis (see heart
    attack)
Crohn's disease 202
Cushing's disease 261

dementia 184
dependence 13
depression **64–73**, 231, 274, 275
dermatitis 282
diabetes insipidus 20, 31, **61–2**
diabetes mellitus 20, 31, **56–9**

diarrhoea 173, 181, 184, 189, 199,
    202–5, 228
diverticulitis 202
dizziness 180
dosages 21, 25
drugs categories/classification **18–20**
    chemical name 21 controlled 22
    essential interactions 23 issues 14
    reduction **24–8** route of
    administration 13 severity 25
    symptomatic 18, **293** trade name 21
dyskinesia 91, 151
(also see Parkinson's disease)
dyspepsia **183–196**

eczema 259, 261, 282, 288
encephalopathy 184
endocrine disease 20, 31, **56–63**
energetics 16, 26
epilepsy 118, 167, **232–241**
euphoria 274

fungal infection 48, 150

gastrointestinal haemorrhage 195, 221
giardiasis 47
glaucoma 233
gout **255–7**

haemorrhoids 205
hay fever 164, 180
(also see rhinitis)
heart attack 28, 60, 137, 138
(also see myocardial infarction)
hepatic failure 119
herpes simplex 50, 51, 52
herpes zoster 51, 52
HIV 50
hormone replacement therapy
    (endocrine disease) 20, 31, **56–63**
hormone replacement therapy
    (female sex hormones) **262–8, 272–6**
human immunovirus (see HIV)
hyperlipidaemia **139–144**
hypertension 29, **98–118**, 122, 167, 272
hyperthyroidism 99
(also see thyrotoxicosis)
hypothyroidism 20, 31, **59–61**

indigestion 221
(also see dyspepsia)
infectious disease **33–54**
infertility 228, 262
influenza 51

insomnia 236
(also see anxiety)

legal considerations 16
life-threatening conditions 21, 26, 31, **55–63**
liver damage 221

manic depression 19, 90, **96–7**
Meniere's disease 180, 233
menopause 262, 272, 273
migraine 19, 99, **221–6**, 237
multiple prescriptions 25
myocardial infarction 273
(also see heart attack)

nasal conditions **148–151**
nausea **180–3**, 196
neuralgia 234
neurosis 64

obesity **74–6**, 199
oedema **118–130**, 233
osteoarthritis 254
osteoporosis 272, 274
otosclerosis 273

pain **210–221**
Parkinson's disease 30, 51, **226–232**
(also see dyskinesia)
peptic ulcer **183–196**, 221
peripheral atherosclerosis 144
peripheral vascular disease **144–7**
pharmacology 11
pituitary tumour 228
pneumonia 200
pre-mentrual tension/syndrome 129, 228, 262, 263
protozoal infection 47
psoriasis 282, **286–8**
psychological disorders 26, **64–97**
psychosis 20, 77, **90–7**, 182, 237
pulmonary oedema 132
(see also oedema)

Raynaud's disease/phenomenon 144
reflux oesophagitis 187
renal disease 129

renal stones 256
respiratory tract infection 44
(also see upper respiratory tract infection)
rheumatoid arthritis 62, 210, 220, 250, 252, 253, 254, 255, 259, 261, 262
rhinitis allergic 148, 151 perennial 148
(also see hay fever)

schizophrenia 20
sexually transmitted disease 31
side-effects **11–13**, 22, 23
skin disease 19, 151
special precautions 22
'stroke' 272, 275
support 26–7
suppression **11–13**, 24 of menstruation 274 of skin disease 282
sustained release 21
systemic lupus erythematosus 48

tendon disease 254
tennis elbow 254, 261
thrombosis 272, 273, 275
'thrush' 47
thyrotoxicosis **61**
(also see hyperthyroidism)
trichomoniasis 47
trigeminal neuralgia 234, 237
tumours 262
(also see cancer)

ulcerative colitis 62, 202, 254, 259
(also see colitis)
upper respiratory tract infection 39
(also see respiratory tract infection)
urinary tract infection 33, 38, 39, 41, 44, 46
urticaria 180

vertigo 180
viral disease 51
vomiting **180–3**, 196

withdrawal 13, 14, 24
(also see drug classification)

DRUG INDEX

Page reference in BOLD type is main entry.

Drugs in CAPITAL LETTERS indicate trade names ie the brand name of the pharmaceutical company which manufactures and markets the product. All these names are therefore Registered Trade Marks.

Drugs not in capital letters indicate chemical names (also known as generic). A single chemical may be marketed by several companies each with their individual brand name.

Names in italics refer to drug groups or general types of drug.
EG TENORMIN – atenolol – *betablocker*

abrasive **289**, 292
absorbent **202**, 203
ACCUPRO **107**
ACE inhibitor **106–107**, 116, 133
acebutolol **101**
ACEPRIL **107**
acetazolamide **119, 234**
acetic acid derivative **249–250**
acetohexamide **57**
ACETOXYL **289**
acetylcysteine **157**
ACEZIDE **107**
ACHROMYCIN **40**
acipimox **142**
ACNEGEL **289**
ACNEGEL FORTE **289**
ACNIDAZIL **289**
acrivastine **152**
ACTIDIL **155**
ACTIFED **160**
ACTIFED COMPOUND **160**
ACTINAC **278**
ACTONORM **184**
ACUPAN **216**
acyclovir **50**
ADALAT **113**
ADALAT RETARD **113**
ADCORTYL **281**
ADCORTYL with GRANEODIN **281**
ADIFAX **76**
ADIZEM **113**
ADIZEM SR **113**
adrenaline **68**, 88, 99, 100, 105, 167, 173, 178
adrenergic neurone blocker **105**
AEROLIN AUTO **172**
AFRAZINE **148**
agar **200**

AGAROL **200**
AKINETON
ALCODERM **284**
alcohol 23, **68**, 71, 74, 75, 91, 192, 214, 217, 229, 286
alcomethasone **278**
ALDACTIDE-25 **125**
ALDACTIDE-50 **125**
ALDACTONE **121**
ALDOMET **99**, 116
ALGICON **184**
alginic acid **187**, 191
ALGITEC **191**
ALIMIX **192**
alkanone **248**
allantoin **278**, 284, 286
ALLEGRON **67**
allopurinol **256**
almasilate **184**
ALMAZINE **80**
ALMODAN **34**
aloin **198**
ALOPHEN **198**
aloxiprin **212**
ALPHA KERI **284**
alpha and betablocker **104–5**

alphablocker **110–112**, 146
ALPHADERM **280**
ALPHOSYL **286**
ALPHOSYL HC **278**
alprazolam **79**
ALRHEUMAT **246**
ALTACITE PLUS **187**
ALU-CAP **184**
ALUDROX **185**
ALUDROX SA **185**
ALUHYDE **185**

ALULINE **256**
aluminium 184, 194
aluminium acetate 208
aluminium chlorhydroxide 280
aluminium hydroxide **169, 184–6**, 187, 188, 194
aluminium oxide **289**
ALUPENT **171**
ALUPRAM **79**
ALUZINE **128**
alverine citrate **188**
amantadine **51–2, 227**
AMBAXIN **35**
ambutonium chloride **185**
AMFIPEN **34**
AMILCO **120**
amiloride 101, 104, **120**, 124
AMILOSPARE **120**
aminoglycosides 129
aminophylline **132, 168–9**
aminoquinoline **252**
amiodarone **55**, 133
amitryptiline 28, 29, **66**
amlodipine 112, **113**
ammonium chloride 157, 159, 160
AMORAM **34**
amoxapine **67**
AMOXIL **34**
amoxycillin **34**
amphetamine 64, 68, 75, 82, 105, 167
amphotericin **48**
ampicillin **34**
amylobarbitone **82**
amylobarbitone sodium **82**
AMYTAL **82**
anabolic steroids **268–9**
ANACAL **208**
anaesthetic 44
(also see local anaesthetic)
ANAFRANIL **67**, 88
analgesic 18, 30, 117, 161, 162, 165, 203, **210–221**, 224, 225, 242, 254, 293
androgen 262, **268–9**
ANDURSIL **185**
ANGETTE **220**
ANGILOL **103**
ANGIOZEM **113**
ANQUIL **92**
antacid 18, 169, **184–7**, 188, 189, 194, 195, 196, 293
antazoline 283
ANTEPSIN **194**
ANTHRANOL **287**

anti-androgen **290**
antibacterial **46–7**, 278, 279, 280, 281, 282, 283, 292
antibiotic 12, 18, **32–54**, 57, 128, 129, 150, 206, 208, 209, **290**, 292
(also see antibacterial)
anticholinergic **148**, 167, 171, **173–4**, 179, **181**, 185, 186, **189–190**, 195, 198, 203, 204, 215, **228**
anticonvulsant 22, 192, **232–241**
antidandruff agent **288**
antidepressant 29, 30, **64–73**, 74, 75, 77, 88, 241 *monoamine oxidase inhibitor* 30, 65, **68–9**, 71, 72, 74, 85, 87, 111, 167, 170, 213, 230, 231, 234 *tetracyclic* **70–1** *tricyclic* 30, 31, 64, **65–8**, 170, 215
antidiabetic 74
antidiuretic hormone **61–2**
antidopaminergic **224–5**, 227
antiemetic 214, 224
antiepileptic 19
antifungal **47–50**, 278, 279, 280, 281, 282, 289
antihistamine **816, 144**, 148, 150, **151–5**, 157, 163, 164, 166, **180–1**, 218, 219, 222, 225, 283, 285
antihypertensive 68, 74, **98–118**
anti-inflammatory **205**, 209, 210, **158–161**, 258
anti-inflammatory agent 19, 192, 207
(also see non-steroidal anti-inflammatory drugs)
antiParkinsonian 30, 68, 97, **226–232**
ANTIPRESSAN **101**
antipruritic 278, 279, **283**, 285
antipsoriatic 278, 279, **286–7**
antipsychotic agent 19, 30, 75, 77, **90–7**, 182
antiseptic 205, 208, 209, **283**, 284, **285**, 288
antispasmodic 185, 187, **188**, 189, 195, 204
antithyroid **61**
antitussive **165**
antiulcer 185, 187, **193–5**
antiviral **50-4**, 227
ANTRADERM **287**
ANTRADERM FORTE **287**
ANTRADERM MILD **287**
ANTURAN **257**
ANUGESIC HC **207**
ANUSOL **205**

ANUSOL HC 207
APISATE 75
APP 185
appetite suppressant **74–6**, 105
APRESOLINE 109
APRINOX 123
APSIFEN 246
APSIFEN F 246
APSIN V.K. 35
APSOLOL 103
APSOLOX 102
AQUADRATE 284
arachis oil 278, 283, 287
ARELIX 129
AROBON 202
ARPICOLIN 228
ARPIMYCIN 42
ARTANE 228
arteriolar dilator 133
ARTHROFEN 246
ARTHROSIN 246
ARTRACIN 247
ARYTHMOL 55
ASACOL 206
ASENDIS 67
ASILONE 185
ASMAVEN 172
ASPAV 211
aspirin 12, 18, 57, 162, 205, 206, 210,
    211–2, 214, 217, 220, 221, 225, 242,
    256
(also see salicylate)
astemizole 152
astringent 205, 208
ATARAX 86
atenolol 101
ATENSINE 79
ATIVAN 77, **80**, 81, 90
ATROMID S 140
atropine 174, 203
ATROVENT 174
ATROVENT FORTE 174
AUGMENTIN 34
auranofin 251
AUREOCORT 281
AUREOMYCIN 40
AVEENO 284
AVEENO OILATED 284
AVENTYL 67
AVOMINE 181
AXID 191
azapropazone 244
azatadine 152

AZT 52

bacampicillin 35
bacitracin 279
bactericide 287
BACTRIM 45
BALNEUM 284
BALNEUM with TAR 286
BALTAR 286
BARATOL 112
barbiturate **81–83**, 90, 217, **236–7**, 238
BARQUINOL HC 278
barrier agent 278
BAXAN 37
BAYCARON 124
B.C.500 with Iron 197
BECLOFORTE 175
beclomethasone 150, 175, 280
BECODISKS 175
BECONASE 150
BECOTIDE 28, **175**
BEDRANOL 103
belladonna 185, **189**, 198
BELLOCARB 189
BENDOGEN 105
bendrofluazide 29, 30, 102, 103, 104,
    117, **123**
BENEMID 257
BENORAL 244
benorylate 244
benperidol 92
benserazide 230, 231
BENTEX 228
BENYLIN 159
BENYLIN DECONGESTANT 159
BENYLIN with CODEINE 159
BENZAGEL 289
benzalkonium 279, 284, **286**, 289
benzamide 95
benzathine penicillin 35
benzhexol 228
benzodiazepine 66, 77, **78–81**, 81, 83,
    86, 192, 235
benzotriazine 244
BENZOYL 5 289
BENZOYL 5 with SULPHUR 289
BENZOYL 10 289
BENZOYL 10 with SULPHUR 289
benzoyl peroxide 279, **289**
benzthiazide 123
benztropine 228
benzylbenzoate 207, 284
BERKAMIL 120

BERKATENS **55, 114**
BERKMYCEN **40**
BERKOLOL **103**
BERKOZIDE **123**
BEROTEC **170**
BETA-ADALAT **101**
beta agonist **132–3, 165–6, 170–3,** 177, 179
betablocker 12, 19, 27, 29, 30, 55, 60, 77, 88, 98, **99–104,** 108, 113, 115, 116, 117, 137, 138, 221, 226
BETACARDONE **103**
BETADINE **288**
betahistine **180**
BETALOC **102**
BETALOC SA **102**
betamethasone **150, 175–6, 207, 259,** 262, **280**
betaxolol 101
bethanidine **105**
BETIM **104**
BETNELAN **259**
BETNESOL **150, 259**
BETNESOL-N **250**
BETNOVATE **280**
BETNOVATE C **281**
BETNOVATE N **281**
BETNOVATE RD **281**
BETNOVATE RECTAL **207**
BEXTASOL **176**
bezafibrate **140–1**
BEZALIP **141**
BEZALIP-MONO **141**
biguanide **58**
bile acid sequestrant **142**
BINOVUM **271**
BIOGASTRONE **194**
BIOPHYLLINE **169**
BIORPHEN **228**
bisacodyl **198**
bismuth **194–5**
bismuth carbonate 185
bismuth oxide 205, 207, 208
bismuth subgallate **205,** 207
bismuth subnitrate 187
bisoprolol **101**
BLOCADREN **104**
BOLVIDON **71**
BRADILAN **142, 145**
bran **199,** 201
BRASIVOL **289**
BREVINOR **271**
BRICANYL **165, 173**

BRICANYL SA **173**
BRITIAZEM **113**
BROCADOPA **230**
BROFLEX **228**
bromazepam **79**
bromocryptine **229**
brompheniramine **152, 158**
BRONCHILATOR **171**
BRONCHODIL **171**
bronchodilator 28, 166, 170, 173, 175, 178, 179, 262
(also see asthma)
bronchorelaxant 164
BROXIL **36**
BRUFEN **246**
BUCCASTEM **183**
buclizine 225
budesonide **150, 175, 281**
bulking agent **58, 76,** 187, 188, **199)200**
bumetanide **126,** 130
buprenorphine **213**
BURINEX **126**
BURINEX K **126**
BUSCOPAN **189**
BUSPAR **83**
buspirone **83**
BUTACOTE **249**
butethamate 167
butobarbitone **82**
butoxyethyl 278
butryptiline **67**
butylphenol **142–3**
butyrophenone **92–3**

CAFADOL **218**
CAFERGOT **222,** 226
caffeine 161, 212, 214, 218, 219, 222
CALABREN **57**
CALADRYL **283**
calamine 278, 279, *283*
calcium 275
calcium antagonist 101, **112–4,** 116, 137
calcium carbonate 185, **186–7**
calcium overload regulator **144–5**
CALENDOLON **283**
calendula *283*
CALMURID **284**
CALMURID HC **280**
CALPOL INFANT **217**
CALPOL SIX PLUS **218**
CALTHOR **35**
CAM **167**
CAMCOLIT **97**

camphor 283
CANESTEN 50
CANESTEN HC 278
CANTIL 190
CAPITOL 286
CAPLENAL 256
CAPOTEN 107
CAPOZIDE 107
CAPRIN 211
captopril 107
CARACE 107
CARBALAX 201
carbamate tranquilliser 87, 212
carbamazepine 96, 235
CARBELLON 189
carbenoxolone 193–4
carbidopa 231
carbimazole 12, 61
carbinoxamine 159
carbocisteine 158
CARBOCORT 278
CARBO-DOME 286
carbonic anhydrase inhibitor 118–9
carboxylic acid derivative 238–9
CARDENE 113
cardiac drugs 20, 31, 55
cardiac glycoside 131–2
CARDIACAP 137
CARDINOL 103
CARDURA 110, 111
carfecillin 35
carmellose 283
carteolol 101
CARTROL 101
CATAPRES 108, 225
CATAPRES PERLONGETS 108
CAVED-S 185
CEANEL Conc 286
CEDILANID 132
CEDOCARD 136
CEDOCARD RETARD 136
cefaclor 37
cefadroxil 37
cefuroxime 37
CELEVAC 76   200   202
central alpha agonist 98–9, 225–6
central nervous system depressant 68,
    214, 238
central nervous system stimulant 74–5
CENTYL 123
CENTYL K 123
cephalexin 37
cephalosporin 37–8, 129

cephradine 38
CEPOREX 37
ceratonia 202
CETAVLON P.C.
cetrimide 283, 284, 286, 288, 289
cetirizine 153
chamomile oil 284
charcoal 189
CHEMOTRIM
chloral hydrate 83, 84
chloramphenicol 278
chlordiazepoxide 66, 79
chlorhexidine 279
chlormethiazole 84–5
chlormezanone 85–6, 218
chlorothiazide 123
chlorpheniramine 153, 163, 164
chlorpromazine 94
chlorpropamide 57
chlorquinaldol 281
chlortetracycline 40, 280, 281
chlorthalidone 101, 102, 124
CHOLEDYL 169
cholestyramine 142
choline magnesium trisalicylate 212
choline theophyllinate 168, 169
ciclacillin 35
cimetidine 191
cinchocaine 207, 208, 285
cineole 161, 162
cinnarizine 144, 180
CINOBAC 41
cinoxacin 41
ciprofloxacin 41
CIPROXIN 41
cisapride 192
citric acid 204
CLARITYN 154
clavulanic acid 34
clemastine 153
clindamycin 290
CLINITAR 286
CLINORIL 248
clioquinol 278, 279, 280, 281
clobazam 79, 235
clobetasol 282
clobetasone 280
clofibrate 139, 140
clomipramine 67
clomocycline 40
clonazepam 235
clonidine 19, 27, 107–8, 116, 225
clopamide 103

CLOPIXOL **93**
clorazepate potassium **79**
clotrimazole **50**, 278, 281
cloxacillin **35**
clozapine **95**
CLOZARIL **95**
coal tar 278, 279, **286–7**
(also see tar)
COBADEX 278
CO-BETALOC **102**
CO-BETALOC SA **102**
CO-CODADRIN **212**
CO-CODAMOL **218**
CODALOX **198**
CODALOX FORTE **198**
CO-DANTHRUSATE **198**
codeine phosphate 156, 158, 160, 161,
   203, 212, **213–4**, 218, 219, 220, 225
CODIS **212**
CO-DYDRAMOL **214**
cod liver oil **284**
COGENTIN **228**
COLESTID **142**
colestipol **142**
COLIFOAM **208**
COLOFAC **188**
COLOGEL **200**
COLPERMIN **189**
COLVEN **188**
COMOX **45**
COMPRECIN **41**
CONCORDIN **68**
CONGESTEZE **152**
CONOVA '30' **271**
COPHOLCO **162**
COPHOLCOIDS **162**
CO-POROXAMOL **214**
CORDARONE-X **55**
CORDILOX **55**, **114**
CORDILOX '160' **114**
CORGARD **102**
CORGARETIC '40' **102**
CORGARETIC '80' **102**
CORLAN **259**
CORO-NITRO **135**
CORTELAN **63**
corticosteroids 27, 28, 31, 50, 57, **62–3**,
   129, **149–150**, 166, **174–6**, 178, 179,
   207–9, 254, **258–262**, **278–283**, 288
cortisone 19, **62–3**, **259**, 262
CORTISTAB **63**, **259**
CORTISYL **63**, **259**
CORWIN **133**

COSURIC **256**
CRADOCAP **288**
crotamiton 278, 283
cough remedies **156–166**, 293
COVERSYL **107**
cyclandelate **145**
cyclizine **181**, 214, 222
CYCLOBRAL **145**
CYCLOGEST **269**
cyclopenthiazide 102, **124**
CYCLO-PROGYNOVA **265**
cyclopyrrolone **86**
CYCLOSPASMOL **145**
cyproheptadine **153**
cytoprotectant **193–5**
cytoproterone **290**
CYTOTET **192**, 195

DAKTACORT 278
DAKTARIN **49–50**
DALMANE **79**
danazol **263**
DANERAL SA **154**
DANOL **263**
DANOL-½ **263**
danthron **198**
DAONIL **58**
DAVENOL **159**
DDAVP **62**
debrisoquine **105**
DECADRON **259**
decarboxylase inhibitor 231
DECASERPYL **114**
DECLINAX **105**
deflatulent 184, 185, 186, 187, 190
DELTACORTISYL **260**
DELTACORTRIL **260**
DELTASTAB **260**
demeclocycline **40**
demulcent 157, 159, 160, 161, 163, 166
DE-NOL **195**
DE-NOLTAB **195**
DEPIXOL **93**
DEPONIT **135**
DERMALEX **284**
DERMOVATE **282**
DERMOVATE NN **282**
DESERIL **224**, 226
desipramine **67**
desmopressin **62**
DESMOSPRAY **62**
desogestrel 271
desoxymethasone **280**, **281**

DETECLO 40
dexamethasone 150, **259**, 262
DEXA-RHINASPRAY 150
dexfenfluramine 76
dextromethorphan 160
dextromoramide **214**, 220
dextropropoxyphene **214**, 220
DF118 **162**, 214
DHC CONTINUS 214
DIABENESE 57
DIAMICRON 58
DIAMOX 119, **234**
DIANETTE 291
DIARREST 203
DIATENSEC 121
diazepam 21, **79**
diazoxide 109
dibenzoxepine 95
diclofenac 245
DICONAL 214
dicyclomine 186, **189**, 203
diethylpropion 74, **75**
DIFLUCAN 48
diflucortolone 281, **282**
diflusinal 212
dugutakus 131
digoxin 12, 129, **132**, 133
dihydrocodeine **162**, 213, **214**, 219, 220
diltiazem 112, **113**
DIMELOR 57
dimenhydrate 181
dimethicone 184, 185, 186, 187, 190, 278, 279
dimethindene 154
DIMOTANE CO 158
DIMOTANE EXPECTORANT 158
DIMOTANE LA 152
DIMOTANE PLUS 153
DIMOTANE PLUS LA 153
DIMOTAPP 159
DIMOTAPP LA 159
dinoestrol 265
DIOCTYL 200
DIODERM 278
DIORYLATE 203
DIOVOL 185
dipipanone **214**, 220
diphenhydramine 157, **159–161**, 219, 283
diphenoxylate 203
diphenylbutylpiperidine 93
diphenylpyraline **154**, 164
diprophylline 168

DIPROBASE 284
DIPROSALIC 281
DIPROSONE 281
DIRYTHMIN SA 55
DISALCID 212
disinfectant 279
DISIPAL 228
disopyramide 55
DISPROL PAED 217
DISTACLOR 37
DISTALGESIC 214
DISTAMINE 253
DISTAQUAINE V-K 36
dithranol 287, **288**
DITHROCREAM 287
DITHROCREAM 2% 287
DITHROCREAM HP 287
DIUMIDE-K CONTINUS **128**
diuretic 12, 22, 29, 30, 57, 98, 106, 108, 115, 116, 117, **118–130** loop (high potency) 120, 122, **125–9**, 130, 133 potassium sparing (low potency) **119–122**, 123, 124, 125, 130, 133 thiazide (medium potency) **122–5**, 130, 133
DIUREXAN 125
DIXARIT 226
docosahexaenoic acid 143
docusate sodium 198, **200**
DOLMATIL 95
DOLOBID 212
DOLOXENE 214
DOLOXENE CO 214
DOMICAL 66
domperidone 181
DOPAMET 99
dopamine 227, 228
dopamine agonist **228–9**
dopamine antagonist 181
dopamine precursor **229–231**
dopaminergic 227
DORMONOCT 79
dothiepin 67
doxazosin 111
doxepin 67
doxycycline 40
doxylamine 219
DOZIC 92
DRAMAMINE 181
DROLEPTAN 19, **92**
droperidol 92
DRYPTAL **128**
DULCOLAX **198**

DUO-AUTOHALER 171
DUOGASTRONE 194
DUOVENT 170
DUPHALAC 201
DUPHASTON 267
DUROMINE 75
DYAZIDE 124
dydrogesterone 267
DYNESE 187
DYSMAN 248
DYSPAMET 191
DYTAC 122
DYTIDE 123

E45 284
EBUFAC 246
ECONACORT 50, 278
econazole 50, 278, 281
ECOSTATIN 50
ECZEDERM 278
ECZEDERM HC 278
EDECRIN 127
EFCORTELAN 278
ELANTAN 136
ELAVIL 66
ELDEPRYL 231
ELECTROLADE 204
electrolyte 203, **204**
ELTROXIN 59
EMCOR 101
EMCOR LS 101
EMESIDE 236
emollient 278, 283, **284**, 285, 286, 287
EMULSIDERM 284
enalapril 107
ENDURON 124
enoxacin 41
EPANUTIN 237
ephedrine 153, 159, **164**, **167**, 168, 178
EPIFOAM 278
EPILIM 239
EPOGAM 285
EQUAGESIC 212
EQUANIL 87
ERALDIN 10
ergot alkaloid 221
ergotamine **221–2**
ERYCEN 42
ERYMAX 43
ERYMAX SPRINKLE 43
ERYTHROCIN 43
ERYTHROMID 43
ERYTHROMID DS 43

erythromycin 42, 290
ERYTHROPED 43
ERYTHROPED A 43
ERYTHROPED FORTE 43
ESBATAL 105
ESIDREX 124
ESKAMEL 291
ESKORNADE 164
ESKORNADE SPANSULE 164
ESTRADERM 265
ESTRAPAK 265
ethacrynic acid 127, 130
ethinyloestradiol 271, 291
ethoheptazine 212
ethosuximide 236
ethynodiol 271, **272**
etodolac 245
eucalyptus 156
EUDEMINE 109
EUGLUCON 58
EUGYNON '30' 271
EUMOVATE 280
EURAX 283
EURAX-Hydrocortisone 278
EVADYNE 67
EVOXIN 181
EXIREL 171
EXOLAN 287
expectorant **157**, 158, 159, 160, 161, 162, 163, 165, 166
EXPULIN 163
EXPURHIN 164

FABAHISTIN 154
FABROL 157
faecal softener 198, **200**
famotidine 191
fanofibrate 140
FASIGYN 47
FAVERIN 70
FECTRIM 45
FEFOL SPANSULE 197
FEFOL-VIT SPANSULE 197
FEFOL Z SPANSULE 197
FELDENE 249
FEMODENE 271
FEMODENE ED 271
FEMULEN 272
fenamate 248
FENBID 246
fenbufen 245
fenfluramine 74, 75, **76**
fenoprofen **245–6**

FENOPRON 245
FENOSTIL RETARD 154
fenoterol 170–1, 178
FENTAZIN 94
FEOSPAN SPANSULE 197
FERFOLIC SV 197
FERGON 197
ferric citrate 196–7
FERROCAP 197
FERROCAP-F '350' 197
FERROCONTIN CONTINUS 197
FERROCONTIN FOLIC CONTINUS
   197
FERROGRAD 197
FERROGRAD C 197
FERROGRAD FOLIC 197
FERROMYN 197
ferrous fumarate 197
ferrous gluconate 197
ferrous succinate 197
ferrous sulphate 197
FERSADAY 1907
FERSAMAL 197
FESOVIT SPANSULE 197
FESOVIT Z SPANSULE 197
fibre 201
FLAGYL 47
flecainide 55
FLEXIN CONTINUS 247
FLORINEF 63
FLOXAPEN 35
FLUANXOL 70
fluclorolone 281
flucloxacillin 35
fluconazole 48
fludrocortisone 62–3
flunisolide 150
flunitrazepam 79
fluocinolone 278–9, 280, 281
flucocinonide 281
fluorcortolone 207, 280
fluoxetine 67
flupenthixol 70, 93
fluphenazine 68, 94
flurandrenolone 280
flurbiprofen 246
fluspirilene 93
fluvoxamine 70
FOLEX '350' 197
folic acid 196, 197
folic acid inhibitor 44–6
FOLICIN 197
FORMULIX 197

FORTAGESIC 216
FORTRAL 216
FORTUNAN 92
framycetin 278
FRAMYCORT 278
frangula 187, 200
FRANOL 167
FRANOL PLUS 167
FRISIUM 79, 235
FROBEN 246
FROBEN SR 246
FRUMAX 128
FRUMIL 120
FRUMIL LS 120
frusemide 103, 120, 133, 127–9, 130
FRUSENE 28, 128
FRUSID 128
FUCIBET 281
FUCIDIN 43
FUCIDIN H 278
FULCIN 49
fungicide 48
FURADANTIN 39
fusidic acid 43, 281
FYBOGEL 199
FYBRANTA 199

GABA analogue 239–240
GALCODINE 161
GALENAMOX 34
GALENPHOL 163
GALFER 197
GALFER LA 197
GALFERVIT 197
GALPSEUD 164
GAMANIL 67
gamolenic acid 285
GASTRESE LA 182
GASTROBID CONTINUS 182
GASTROCOTE 187
GASTROFLUX 182
GASTROMAX 182
GASTRON 188
GASTROZEPIN 190
GAVISCON 188
GELCOSAL 286
GELCOTAR 286
GELUSIL 185
gemfibrozil 141
GENISOL 286
gentamicin 279
GENTICIN HC 279
gestodene 271

GIVITOL **197**
glibenclamide **57**
GLIBINESE **58**
glicazide **58**
glipizide **58**
gliquidone **58**
glucocorticoid **62–3**
GLUCOPHAGE **59**
glucose 204
GLURENORM **58**
glycerides 284
glycerol 284
glyceryl trinitrate **135–5**, 138
gold salt **250–1**, 254
grain fibre **199**
gramicidin 281, 282
GREGODERM **279**
griseofulvin 48
GRISOVIN **49**
guaiphenesin **158**, 160, 165
guanethidine **105**
GUANOR **157**
guar gum **58**
GUAREM **58**
GUARINA **58**
GYNO-DAKTARIN **50**
GYNOPEVARYL **50**

H2 blocker **190–1**, 193, 195
HAELAN **280**
HAELAN-C **280**
HAELAN TAPE **280**
HAELAN-X **280**
HALCIDERM **282**
halcinonide **282**
HALCION **80**
HALDOL **83**
HALF INDERAL LA **103**
HALOPERIDOL **92**
HARMOGEN **266**
HEMINEVRIN **85**
heparin 12
heparinoid **205**, 208
heroin 213
hexachlorophane 208, 284, 289
hexamine **46**
HEXOPAL **145**
HEXOPAL FORTE **145**
HIPRAL **47**
HISMANAL **152**
HISTALIX **160**
histamine analogue **180**
HISTRYL SPANSULE **154**

HMG CoA Reductase inhibitor **143–4**
homatropine 185
hormone replacement therapy 22
(also see sex hormones)
hormones **52–63** antidiuretic **61–2** sex
   (see sex hormones) thyroid **59–61**
HORMONIN **266**
HUMIDERM **284**
hyaluronidase 205
hydantoin **237–8**
hydralazine 133, **109**
hydrating agent 279, 280
HYDRENOX **125**
HYDROCAL **279**
hydrochlorothiazide **99**, 101, 102, 103,
   104, 107, 120, 121, **124**
hydrocortisone 50, **62–3**, **207–8**, **259**,
   262, **281**, 282
hydrocortisone-butyrate 281
HYDROCORTISTAB **63**, **259**, **279**
HYDROCORTISYL **63**
HYDROCORTONE **63**, **259**
hydroflumethazide **125**
HYDROMET **99**
HYDROMOL **284**
HYDROSALURIC **124**
hydrotalcite **187**
hydroxychloroquine **252**
5-hydroxytryptamine reuptake
   inhibitor **70**
hydroxyzine **86**
HYGROTON **124**
HYGROTON K **124**
hyoscine **181**, 189
HYPERTANE **120**
hypnotic 88
(also see tranquillisers)
hypoglycaemic agents **56–9**, 68, 176
HYPON **121**
hypotensive agents 12, 19, 30, **98–118**,
   122, 128
HYPOVASE **110**, **146**
HYTRIN **110**, **111**

ibuprofen **246**
idoxuridine **52**
IDURIDIN **51**
ILOSONE **43**
IMBRILON **247**
IMDUR **136**
imidazole **49–50**
iminostilbene **96**, **234–5**
imipramine 64, 66, **67**

IMODIUM 203
immunosuppressant 106, 254
IMMUNOVIR 52
IMPERACIN 40
indapamide 125
INDERAL 60, 88, **103**
INDERAL LA 103
INDERETIC 103
INDEREX 103
INDOCID 247
INDOLAR SR 247
indole 247–8
INDOMETHACIN 247
INDOMOD 247
indoramin 111–2
inosine 52–3
inositol 145
INNOVACE 107
insulin 12, 31, **56–7**, 140
INTAL 27, **177**, 178, 179
INTAL Compound 177
INTEGRIN 87, 94
IONAMIN 75
IONAX 289
IONIL T 286
ipecacuanha 198
IPRAL 45
ipratropium 148, 174
iprindole 67
iron **196–7**
ISMELIN 105
ISMO 136–7, 138
isoaminile 165
ISO-AUTOHALER 171
isocarboxazid 69
isoetharine 171
ISOGEL 199
ISOKET RETARD 136
isometheptene 224
isoprenaline 55, **171**, 177
ISORDIL 136
ISORDIL TEMBIDS 136
isosorbide dinitrate 133, **136**
isosorbide monomitrate 28, **136–7**
ISOTRATE 137
ispaghula husk 188, **199**
isradipine 112, **113**
ISTIN 113
itraconazole 48

JUNIFEN 246

KALSPARE 124

KALTEN 101
KAMILLOSAN 284
KAODENE 203
kaolin **202**, 203, 284
KAOPECTATE 202
KEFLEX 37
KELFIZINE 44
KEMADRIN 228
keratolytic 278, 280, 281, 284, 286,
    290, 291, 292
KERI 284
KERLONE 101
KEST 202
ketoconazole 49–50
ketoprofen 246
ketotifen 156, 176
KIDITARD 55
KINIDIN DURULES 55
KOLANTICON 186

labetalol 105
LABOPRIN 212
LABROCOL 105
lactic acid 280, 284
LACTICARE 284
lactulose 201
LADROPEN 35
laevulose 204
lanatoside-C 132
lanolin 285
LANOXIN-125 132
LANOXIN 132
LANOXIN-PG 132
LARACTONE 121
LARAFLEX 246
LARATRIM 45–6
LARGACTIL 19, 24, 30, 77, **94**
LARODOPA 230
LASIKAL 128
LASILACTONE 122
LASIPRESSIN 103
LASIX 128
LASIX+K 128
LASMA 169
LASONIL 205
LASORIDE 120
lauromacrogol 208
laxatives 20, 57, **198–202**, 293
LAXOBERAL 199
LEDERCORT 260, **281**
LEDERFEN 245
LEDERMYCIN 40
LEJFIBRE 199

LENIUM **288**
LENTIZOL **66**
LERGOBAN **154**
levodopa 68, **230–1**
levonorgestrel **265**, 271, 272
levorphanol 220
LEXOTAN **79**
LEXPEC WITH IRON **196**
LEXPEC WITH IRON-M **197**
LIBANIL **58**
LIBRIUM **79**
licorice 185, 187
LIDIFEN **246**
lignocaine 207, 208
LIMBITROL '5' **66**
LIMBITROL '10' **66**
LINGRAINE **222**, 226
liothyronine **59**
LIPANTIL **140**
lipid lowering agents **138–144**
LIPOBASE **284**
liquid paraffin **200**, **284**
lisinopril **107**
LISKONUM **97**
LITAREX **97**
lithium 19, 22, 90, **96–7**, 122, 126
LOBAK **218**
local anaesthetic 68, 186, 207, 208, 209, 278, **285**
LOCOBASE **284**
LOCOID **281**
LOCOID C **281**
LODINE **235**
LOESTRIN '20' **271**
LOESTRIN '30' **271**
lofepramine **67**
LOGYNON **271**
LOGYNON ED **271**
LOMOTIL **203**
LONITEN **110**
loperamide **203**
LOPID **141**
loprazolam **79**
LOPRESOR **102**
LOPRESOR SR **102**
LOPRESORETIC **102**
loratadine **154**
lorazepam **80**
lormetazepam **80**
LOSEC **193**, 195
LOTRIDERM **281**
LOTUSSIN **160**
LOXAPAC **95**

loxapine **95**
LSD (lysergic acid diethylamide) 223
lubricant **200**
LUDIOMIL **70**
LURSELLE **143**
lymecycline **40**
lypressin **62**
lysine 212
lysuride 229

MAALOX **186**
MAALOX PLUS **186**
MAALOX TC **186**
MACRODANTIN **39**
macrolide **42–3**
MADOPAR '62, 5' **230**
MADOPAR '125' **231**
MADOPAR '250' **231**
MADOPAR CR **231**
magaldrate **187**
MAGNAPEN **35**
magnesium 184
magnesium alginate 184
magnesium carbonate 184, 185, **187**, 188, 189
magnesium chloride 283
magnesium hydroxide 184, 185, 186, **187**, 189
magnesium oxide 185, 186, 187
magnesium sulphate **201**
magnesium trisilicate 185, **187**, 188, 189, 194
MALIX **58**
MANEVAC **199**
MANTADINE **51, 227**
MAOI (see antidepressants)
maprotiline **70**
marine triglycerides **143**
MARPLAN **69**
MARVELON **271**
mast cell stabiliser 28, **149**, 150, **156**, 176–8, 179
MAXEPA **143**
MAXOLON **181**
MAXOLON SR **181**
mazindol 74, **75**
MCR-50 **137**
mebeverine **188**
mebhydroline **154**
medazepam **80**
MEDIHALER-DUO **171**
MEDIHALER-ERGOTAMINE **222**
MEDIHALER-ISO **171**

MEDISED 218
MEDOMET 99
MEDRONE 259, 280

medroxyprogesterone 267
mefruside 124
MEGACLOR 40
MELLERIL 19, 94
MENOPHASE 265
MENZOL 268
menthol 156, 159, 160, 161, 162, 163
mepenozalate 190
meprobamate 87, 123, 212
meptazinol 215
MEPTID 215
mequitazine 154
MERBENTYL 189
MERCILON 271
mesalazine 206
mesterolone 269
mestranol 265
METENIX 124
METERFOLIC 197
metformin 59
methadone 214, 220
methionine 218
methixene 228
methocarbamol 212
methoserpidine 114
methotrimeprazine 94
methyclothiazide 124
methylcellulose 76, 200, 202
methylcysteine 158
methyldopa 98, 99, 116
methylphenobarbitone 236
methylprednisolone 259, 262, 280
methysergide 222–4
metoclopramide 181, 182, 225
metolazone 124
metoprolol 102
METOROS 102
METOROS LS 102
METOSYN 281
METOX 182
METROLYL 47
metronidazole 47
mexiletine 55
MEXITIL 55
mianserin 71
miconazole 50, 278, 289
MICROGYNON '30' 271
MICRONOR 272
MICROVAL 272

MICTRAL 42
MIDAMOR 120
MIDRID 224, 226
MIGRALEVE 225, 226
MIGRAVESS 225, 226
MIGRAVESS FORTE 225
MIGRIL 222, 226
MILDISON LIPOCREAM 279
milk solids 186
mineralocorticoid 62–3
MINOCIN 40
MINOCIN '50' 40
minocycline 40
MINODIAB 58
minoxidil 110
MINTEC 189
MINULET 271
misoprostol 192
MOBIFLEX 249
MODECATE 94
MODITEN 94
MODRASONE 277
MODUCREN 104
MODURET-25 120
MODURETIC 125
MOGADON 80, 88
moisturiser 285
(also see emollients)
MOLIPAXIN 72
MONIT 137
MONIT LS 137
monoalkylolamide 287
monoamine oxidase inhibitor (see
    antidepressants)
monoamine oxidase-B inhibitor 231
(also see antidepressants for
    monoamine oxidase inhibitor)
MONO-CEDOCARD 137
MONOCOR 101
MONOTRIM 45
MONOVENT 173
MONOVENT SA
MORHULIN 284
morphine 11, 156, 204, **214–5**, 220
MORSEP 284
MOTILIUM 181
MOTIPRESS 68
MOTIVAL 68
MOTRIN 246
MST CONTINUS 214
MUCAINE 186
MUCODYNE 158
MUCOGEL 186

mucolytic **157**, 166
MYCARDOL **137**
MYOCRISIN **251**
MYSOLINE **238**
MYSTECLIN **41**

nabumetone **248**
NACTON **190**
MACTON FORTE **190**
nadolol **102**
naftidrofuryl oxalate **146**
NALCROM **156**
nalidixic acid **42**
NAPROSYN **246**
naproxen **246–7**
NARDIL **68**
NARPHEN **215**
nasal sprays **148–151**, 293
NATRILIX **125**
NATUDERM **284**
NAVIDREX **124**
NAVIDREX K **124**
NAVISPARE **124**
nedocromil **177–8**
nefopam **215–6**
NEGRAM **42**
NEOCON 1/35 **271**
neogest **272**
NEO-MEDRONE **280**
NEO-MERCAZOLE **61**
neomycin 150, 208, 279, 280, 281, 282
NEO-NACLEX **123**
NEO-NACLEX K **123**
NEPHRIL **125**
NERICUR **289**
NERISONE **281**
NERISONE FORTE **2892**
NEULACTIL **94**
nicardipine 112, **113**
nicofuranose **142, 145**
nicotinic acid derivative **142, 145**
nicotinyl alcohol **145**
nifedipine 101, 112, **113**
NIFEREX **197**
NILSTIM **76**
NITRADOS **80**
nitrate 25, **134–7**, 138
nitrazepam **80**
NITROCONTIN CONTINUS **135**
nitrofuran **38–9**
nitrofurantoin **39**
nitroimidazole **47**
NITROLINGUAL **135**

nizatidine **191**
NIZORAL **50**
NOBRIUM **80**
NOCTEC **84**
non-benzodiazepine tranquilliser **83**
non-steroidal antiflammatory drugs 210,
  220, **242–250**, 254, 255, 262
non-thiazide diuretic **125**
NORDOX **40**
norethisterone 266, **268**, 271, 272
NORGESTON **272**
norgestrel 271, **272**
NORIDAY **272**
NORIMIN **271**
NORINYL-1 **271**
NORMACOL **200**
NORMACOL PLUS **200**
NORMAX **198**
NORMETIC **121**
NORMISON **80**
nortryptiline **67**
NORVAL **71**
NOZINAN **94**
NSAID's (see non-steroidal
  antiflammatory drugs)
NUELIN **169**
NUELIN SA **169**
NULACIN **186**
NUMOTAC **171**
NUPERCAINAL **285**
NU-SEALS Aspirin **211**
NUTRAPLUS **284**
NYSTADERMAL **281**
NYSTAFORM HC **279**
NYSTAN **48**
nystatin **48**, 279, 280, 281, 282

oat bran 189
oat fraction **284**
oestradiol **265**, 266
oestriol 265, **266**,
oestrogen 56, 262, **264–6**, 269, 273,
  274, 291
(also see sex hormones)
oestrone 266
ofloxacin **42**
OILATUM EMOLLIENT **284**
OLBETAM **142**
olsalazine **206**
opiate 68, 90, 158, 159, 160, *161–4*, 166,
  203, 204, 205, 211, 212, **213–5**, 216,
  218, 219, 220, 225
opiate agonist-antagonist **215–7**

OPILON 146
OPREN 10
OPTIMINE 152
ORABASE 283
ORABET 59
ORAHESIVE 283
oral contraceptive 13, 39, 48, 56, 57, 234, 237, **269–272**, 273, 274, 291, 292
(also see sex hormones, oestrogen, progestogen)
ORAP 93
ORBENIN 35
orciprenaline 171
orphenadrine 30, 31, **228**
ORTHO-DINOESTROL 265
ORTHO-GYNEST 266
ORTHO-NOVIN 1/50 271
ORUDIS 246
ORUVAIL 246
osmotic laxative 201
OTRIVINE 148–9
OVESTIN 266
OVRAN 271
OVRAN '30' 271
OVRANETTE 271
OVYSMEN 271
OXANID 80
oxatomide 154
oxazepam 80
oxazine 72–3
oxethazine 186
oxicam 249
oxpentifylline 147
oxprenolol 102
oxymetazoline 148
OXYMYCIN 40
oxypertine 87, 94
OXYPRENIX 102
oxytetracycline 40, 279

PALAPRIN FORTE 212
PALDESIC 217
PALFIUM 213
PAMETON 218
PANADOL 218
PANALEVE 217
PANOXYL 289
PANOXYL AQUAGEL 289
papayeretum 211
papaverine 163, 164, 185
paracetamol 18, 29, 30, 53, 117, 161, 162, 165, 210, 214, 216, **217–220**, 221, 224, 225

paracetamol antidote 218
PARACODOL 219
paraffin liquid **200**, 284, 285 soft 284, 285
PARAHYPON 219
PARAKE 219
PARAMAX 225, 226
PARAMOL 162, **219**
PARDALE 219
PARLODEL 229
PARMID 182
PARNATE 69
PARSTELIN 69
partial beta agonist 132–3
PAVACOL-D 163
PAXALGESIC 214
PAXOFEN 246
PECRAM 132, 168
PENBRITIN 34
penbutolol 103
PENDRAMINE 2563
penicillamine 253, 254
penicillin 33–6, 37
penicillin derivative 252–3
penicillin V 35
PENIDURAL 35
pentaerythritol tetranitrate 137
PENTASA 206
pentazocine 216–7
PEPCID PM 191
peppermint oil 161, 187, **188–9**
PERCUTOL 135
PERIACTIN 153
pericyazine 94
perindopril 107
peripheral and cerebral activator 145–6
perphenazine 66, 67, **94**
PERTOFRAN 67
Peru balsam 205, 207, 208
PETROLAGAR N 200
PEVARYL 50
PEVARYL TC 281
PHASAL 97
phenacetin 210, 220
phenazocine 215, 220
phenazopyridine 44
phenelzine 69
PHENERGAN 154
phenethicillin 36
phenindamine 154
pheniramine 154
phenobarbitone 238
phenolpthalein **198**, 200, 201

phenothiazine 30, 67, 68, 69, 77, **93–4**, 182–3
phenothiazine-like 87
PHENSEDYL **160**
phentermine 74, **75**
phenylacetic acid **245**
phenylbutazone 244, **249**
phenylephrine 159, 161, 171, 207
phenylpropanolamine 159, **164**
phenytoin sodium 72, **237**
pholcodine 159, **162**
PHOLCOMED-D **163**
PHOLCOMED-D FORTE **163**
PHYLLOCONTIN **132**
PHYLLOCONTIN CONTINUS 132, **168**
PHYLLOCONTIN FORTE 132, **169**
PHYSEPTONE **214**
pimozide **93**
pindolol **103**
pine oil 161
pinenozalate **190**
piperazine oestrone sulphate **266**
PIPORTIL DEPOT **94**
pipothiazine **94**
PIPTAL **190**
PIPTALIN **190**
pirbuterol **171**
pirenzepine **190**
piretanide **129**, 130
PIRITON **153**
PIRITON SPANDETS **153**
piroxicam **249**
PITRESSIN **62**
pivampicillin **36**
pivmecillinam **36**
pizotifen **224**
PLAQUENIL **252**
PLATET **211**
platinum 16
PLESMET **197**
poldine **190**
poloxamer 198
POLYCROL **186**
POLYCROL FORTE **186**
polyene antibiotic **48**
polyethylene granules **289**
polymyxin B 208, 279
POLYTAR **287**
POLYTAR EMOLLIENT **286**
POLYTAR PLUS **287**
polythiazide **125**
PONDERAX Pacaps **76**

PONDOCILLIN **36**
PONSTAN 242, **248**
potassium bicarbonate 184, 194
potassium chloride 118, 123, 124, 126, 128, 129, 130, 203, 204
potassium hydroxyquinoline sulphate 279, 289
povidone-iodine **288**
PRAGMATAR **287**
pramoxine 207, 278
PRAXILENE **146**
prazosin **110–1**, 133, **146**
PRECORTISYL **260**
PRECORTISYL FORTE **260**
PREDENEMA **208**
PREDFOAM **208**
PREDNESOL **260**
prednisolone 12, 28, **62–3**, 179, **208–9**, **260**, 262
(also see corticosteroids)
prednisone **260**
PREDSOL **208**
PREFERID **281**
PREFIL **76**
PREGADAY **197**
PREGNAVITE Forte F **197**
PREMARIN **266**
PREMPAK-C **266**
PREPULSID **192**
PRESCAL **113**
PRESTIM **104**
PRIADEL **97**
PRIMALAN **154**
primidone **238**
PRIMOLUT N **268**
PRIMPERAN **182**
PRO-ACTIDIL **155**
PRO-BANTHINE **190**
probucol **143**
procainamide **55**
PROCAINAMIDE DURULES **55**
prochlorperazine **94**, 183
PROCTOFIBE **199**
PROCTOFOAM HC **208**
PROCTOSEDYL **208**
procyclidine **228**
PROGESIC **245**
progesterone **268**
(also see progestogen)
progestogen 56, 265, **266–8**, 269, 272, 273
(also see progesterone)
PROGYNOVA 265

prokinetic 191–2
promazine 94
promethazine 86, 154, 160, 181, 218
PROMINAL 236
PRONDOL 67
PRONESTYL 55
PROPADERM 280
PROPADERM A 280
PROPAIN 219
propanolol 103
propantheline 190
propafenone 55
propionic acid 245–7
prostaglandin analogue 192
PROTHIADEN 30, 31, 67
proton pump inhibitor 193
protryptiline 68
PRO-VENT 169
PROVERA 267
PRO-VIRON 269
PROZAC 67
pseudoephedrine 152, 153, 155, 158,
    160, 163, 164–5
PSDRADRATE 287
PSORIDERM 287
PSORIGEL 287
PSORIN 287
psychoactive agents 64–97
PULMADIL 172
PULMICORT 175
PULMICORT LS 175
pyranocarboxylate 245
pyrazone 248–9
pyrimidinedione 238
PYROGASTRONE 194

QUESTRAN 142
QUESTRAN A 142
quinalbarbitone 82
quinapril 107
quinidine 55
quinine 252
QUINOCORT 279
QUINODERM 289
QUINODERM with
    HYDROCORTISONE 279
quinolone 41-2

RABRO 187
ramipril 107
ranitidine 191
RASTINON 58
Rauwolfia alkaloid 114–5, 116

R.B.C. 283
REDEPTIN 93
reflux suppressant 184, 187–8, 194
REGULAN 200
REHIDRAT 204
RELIFLEX 248
REMNOS 80
reproterol 171
reserpine 114
resorcinol 291
RESTANDOL 269
RETCIN 43
RETIN-A 291
RETROVIR 54
REVANIL 229
RHEUMOX 244
RHINOCORT 150
RHUMALGAN 245
RIDAURA 251
rimiterol 171
RINATEC 148
RIVOTRIL 235
ROBAXISAL FORTE 212
ROHYPNOL 79
RONICOL 145
RONICOL TIMESPAN 145
ROTER 187
RUSYDE 128
RYBARVINRYNACROM 149
RYNACROM COMPOUND 149
RYTHMODAN 55

SABIDAL SR 169
SABRIL 240
saccharine 204
SALAZOPYRIN 207
SALAZOPYRIN EN 207, 254
SALBULIN 172
salbutamol 172, 175
SALBUVENT 172
salicylate 57, 205–6, 209, 210–2, 214,
    220, 225
(also see aspirin)
salicylate-paracetamol 244
salicylate-sulphonamide 206–7, 209, 254
salicylic acid 210, 281, 286, 287
salsalate 212
SALURIC 123
SALZONE 217
SANOMIGRAN 224, 226
SAVENTRINE 55
SCHERIPROCT 208
SCOPODERM 181

SECADREX **83**
SECONAL **82**
SECTRAL **101**
SECURON **55, 114**
SECURON SR **114**
sedative 23, 64, 71, *83–6*, 88, 90, 117, 205
(also see tranquillisers)
selegiline 30, 81, **231**
selenium **288**
SELEXID **36**
SELSUN **288**
SEMI-DAONIL **58**
SEMPREX **152**
SENNA TABLETS **199**
sennosides **198**, 199
SENOKOT **199**, **202**
SENTIAL **279**
SENTIAL E **284**
SEPTRIN 44, **45–6**
SERC **180**
SERENACE 19, 90, **98**
serotonin antagonist **222–3**
serotoninergic **75–6**
SERPASIL **114**
SERPASIL ESIDREX **115**
sex hormones **262–276**
silicic acid 284
SILOXYL **186**
SIMECO **186**
simvastatin **144**
SINEMET 'ls' **231**
SINEMET '110' 30, 31, **231**
SINEMET '275' **231**
SINEMET 'PLUS' **231**
SINEQUAN **67**
SINTISONE **260**
skin protectant **283**
sleeping tablets – hypnotics (see tranquillisers)
SLO-PHYLLIN **170**
SLOW-PREN **102**
SLOW-TRASICOR **102**
sodium 184, 204, 217
sodium alginate 194
SODIUM AMYTAL **82**
sodium aurothiomalate **251**
sodium bicarbonate 185, 187, 188, 201, 203
sodium chloride 203, **204**, 279, 284, 285
sodium citrate 157, 159, 160, 203
sodium cromoglycate **149**, **156**, **177**

sodium fusidate **43**, 278
sodium picosulphate **199**
sodium pyrrolidone **284**
sodium valproate **239**
SOLIS **79**
SOLPADOL **219**
SOLPRIN **212**
SOMINEX **86**
SOMNITE **80**
SONERYL **82**
SONI-SLO **136**
soothing 207, 208, 209
SORBICHEW **136**
SORBID SA **136**
SORBITRATE **136**
SOTACOR **103**
sotalol **103**
SOTAZIDE **103**
soya oil **284**, 286
squalane **284**
SPARINE **94**
SPASMONAL **188**
SPIRETIC **121**
SPIROCTAN **121**
SPIROLONE **121**
spironolactone **121–2**, 125
SPIROSPARE **121**
SPORANOX **48**
STABILLIN V-K **36**
STAFOXIL **35**
stanozolol **269**
STAPHLIPEN **35**
starch **202**
STELAZINE 90, **94**, **183**
STEMETIL 29, 30, **94**, 117, **183**
sterculia **76**, **200**
steroids (see corticosteroids)
STIEDEX **281**
STIEDEX LP **280**
STIEDEX LP N **280**
STIEMYCIN **290**
stilboestrol **266**
stimulant laxative **198–9**, 200, 201, 202
STROMBA **269**
STUGERON **180**
STUGERON FORTE **144**
succinimide **238**
sucralfate **194**
sucrose 203
SUDAFED **165**
SUDAFED-CO **165**
SUDAFED PLUS **155**
SUDAFED SA **165**

SUDOCREM 284
sulfametopyrazine 44
sulindac 248
sulphacarbamide 44
sulphamethoxazole 45–6
sulphasalazine 207, 254
sulphinpyrazone 256–7
sulphonamide 44, 46, 206
sulphur 278, 280, 287, 288, 291
sulpiride 95
SULPITIL 95
SUREM 80
SURGAM 247
SURMONTIL 68
SUSCARD BUCCAL 135
SUSTAC 135–6
SUSTAMYCIN 40
SYMMETREL 51, 227
sympathomimetic 68, 74, 105, **148–9**,
    150, 152, 153, 155, 158, 159, 160, 161,
    163, **164–5**, 166, **167–8**, 171, 178, 179,
    207, 215, 224, 241
SYNALAR 1:10 278
SYNALAR 1:4 280
SYNALAR 281
SYNALAR GEL 281
SYNALAR C 281
SYNALAR N 281
SYNDOL 219
SYNFLEX 247
SYNOGIST 287
SYNPHASE 271
SYNTARIS 150
SYNTOPRESSIN 62
SYRAPRIM 45
SYTRON 197

T GEL 287
TAGAMET 183, **191**
talampicillin 36
talc 284
TALPEN 36
TAMBOCOR 55
TAMPOVAGAN 266
tar 286, 288
(also see coal tar)
TARCORTIN 279
TARIVID 42
TAVEGIL 153
TEGRETOL **96**, 235
temazepam 80
TEMGESIC 213
TENAVOID 123

TENIF 101
TENORET 101
TENORETIC 101
TENORMIN 101
TENORMIN LS 29, 30, **101**, 117, 118
tenoxicam 249
TENSIUM 79
TENUATE DOSPAN 75
terazosin 111
terbutaline 172
TERCODA 161
terfenadine 154
TERONAC 75
terpin 161, 163
TERPOIN 161
TERRA-CORTRIL 279
TERRA-CORTRIL NYSTATIN 279
TERRAMYCIN 40
TERTROXIN 59
testosterone 268, **269**
TETRABID 41
TETRACHEL 40
tetracyclic antidepressant **70–1**
tetracycline **39–41**, 290
TETRALYSAL 40
thalidomide 10
THEO-DROX 169
THEO-DUR 170
theophylline **132**, 162, 167, 168,
    169–170
THEPHORIN 154
thiazide 99, 101, 102, 103, 104, 107, 115
    120, 121, **122–5**, 130
(also see diuretics)
thioridazine 94
thioxanthene **69–70**, 92
THOVALINE 284
thymoxamine 146
thyroid hormone 31, **59–61**
thyroxine **59–60**
tiaprofenic acid 247
TIEMPE 45
TILADE 177
TILDIEM 113
TIMODINE 279
timolol 104
tinidazole 47
TINSET 154
tocainide 55
TOFRANIL 64, 67
TOLANASE 58
tolazamide 58
tolbutamide 58

TOLECTIN **250**
TOLERZIDE **103**
tolmetin **250**
TONOCARD **55**
TOPAL **188**
TOPICYCLINE **290**
TOPILAR **281**
TORBETOL **289**
TORECAN **183**
TOTAMOL **101**
tramazoline 150
TRANCOPAL **86**
trancylpromine 69
TRANDATE **105**
tranquilliser 19, 20, 29, 30, 64, 73,
    77–97, 123, 212, 214, 218
TRANSIDERM-NITRO **135**
TRANXENE **79**
TRASICOR **102**
TRASIDREX **102**
trazodone 72
TREMONIL **228**
TRENTAL **147**
tretiniub **291**
TRI-ADCORTYL **281**
triamcinolone 50, **260**, 262, **281**
TRIAMCO **124**
triamterene **122**, 123, 124, 128
triazole **48–9**
triazolam 80
triazolopyridine **71–2**
TRICICATRIN **279**
tricyclic antidepressant (see
    antidepressants)
triethylperazine **113**
trifluoperazine 69, **94**
trifluperidol 93
TRILISATE **212**
TRILUDAN **154**
TRILUDAN FORTE **154**
trimeprazine **155**
trimethoprim **45**
trimipramine 68
TRIMOPAN **45**
TRIMOVATE **280**
TRINORDIOL **271**
TRINOVUM **271**
TRINOVUM ED **271**
TRIPERIDOL **93**
tripotassium dicitratobismuthate **195**
triprolidine **154**, 160
TRIPTAFEN **66**
TRIPTAFEN M **67**

TRISEQUENS **266**
TRITACE **107**
TROPIUM **79**
TRYPTIZOL **66**
TUINAL **82**
TYLEX **220**

ULTRABASE **284**
ULTRADIL **280**
ULTRANUM **280**
ULTRAPROCT **207**
UNGUENTUM **284**
UNIFLU AND GREGOVITE C **161**
UNIGEST **186**
UNIMYCIN **40**
UNIPHYLLIN CONTINUS **132, 170**
UNIROID **208**
UNISOMNIA **80**
UNIVER **114**
urea 219, 280, **284**, 287
URIBEN **42**
uricosuric 255, **256–7**
UROMIDE **44**
UTICILLIN **35**
UTOVLAN **268**

VALENAC **245**
VALIUM 21, 28, 29, 77, **79**, 83, 89
VALLERGAN **154**
VALLERGAN FORTE **154**
VALOID **181**
VALROX **247**
VASCARDIN **136**
VASETIL **120**
vasodilator **108–112**, 116, 133
(also see venodilator, arteriolar
    dilator)
vasopressin 31
V-CIL-K **36**
venodilator 133
VENTIDE **175**
VENTODISKS **172**
VENTOLIN **172**
VENTOLIN CR **172**
viloxacine 73
VIVALAN **73**
VELOSEF **38**
VERACTIL
verapamil 55, 112, **114**
VERTIGON **183**
VIBRAMYCIN **40**
VIBROCIL **148**
VIDOPEN **35**

VIOFORM-Hydrocortisone 279
VIRUDOX 52
VISCLAIR 158
VISKALDIX 103
VISKEN 103
VISTA-METHASONE 150
VISTA-METHASONE N 150
vitamin A derivative 291, 292
vitamin A 284
vitamin B 197
vitamin B6 230, 253
vitamin C 161, 197
vitamin E 146
VOLMAX 172
VOLRAMAN 245
VOLTAROL 245
VOLTAROL RETARD 245
    WARFARIN 12
WELLDORM 84
wool alcohol 284
wool fat 284, 285

xamoterol 133
XANAX 79
xanthine 132, 133, **147**, 161, **162**,
168–170, 179, 212, 214, 218, 219, 220,
    222
xanthine oxidase inhibitor 255–6
XANTHOMAX 256
XIPAMIDE 125
XYLOMETAZOLINE 149
xyloproct 208

ZADITEN **156**, **176**, 179
ZADSTAT 47
ZANTAC 183, **191**, 193
ZARONTIN 236
ZESTRIL 107
zidovudine 52
ZIMOVANE 86
zinc 196, 197
zinc oxide 205, 207, 208, 284
ZINERYT 290
ZINNAT 37
ZIRTEK 153
ZOCOR 144
zopiclone 86
ZOVIRAX 51
zuclopenthixol 93
ZYLORIC 256